Tools to Beat Counting Sheep
And Other Helpful Facts About Sleep

By Chayse Leith

Copyright © 2023 Chayse Leith
All rights reserved.
ISBN-13: 9798378326778

Table of Contents

Preface	4
Chapter One - What is Sleep?	8
Chapter Two - Sleep and the Brain	20
Chapter Three - Hormones and Sleep	32
Chapter Four - Sleep and Physical Health	46
Chapter Five - Sleep and Mental Health	63
Chapter Six - How to Improve Your Sleep	81
Bed Times and Waking Times	84
Bedtime Routine	86
Must do's and Counting Wins	93
Brain Dump	95
Gratefulness Check	97
Doodle Space	99
Sleep Hygiene Checks	101
Loving-Kindness	102
Today's Quotable	105
Chapter Seven - References	107

Preface

As the title proclaims, this book exists to serve you in your endeavours of getting a better night's sleep. The idea came to me mostly through literally hundreds of meetings with people looking to better their health, and feeling like sleep was this ethereal space that needed pixie dust and prayers to achieve fully (or at least some expensive exotic herb or chronic medication). Where in 90% of cases; which is a made up statistic, it can be a far less taxing skill to develop and involves next to no magic.

Sleep is also a commonly overlooked lifestyle factor that sits at the root of many of our physical and mental health woes. The more we are aware of how it may impact us the easier it will be to make moves to improve it. Yes this can still take some time and a little effort, but as with most things the first few steps are hard - once the ball is rolling you will be doing it with your eyes closed (pun most definitely intended).

In this book I have tried my best to explain some of the science behind sleep in easy to digest ways. I think we all should have access to understanding these things without needing to do a degree or learn a new language just to read a book about it. Occasionally you might see a number in brackets within the text; like this one (1), these exist to help direct you around chapter seven, which is just a list of papers containing more information. If you want to learn more about the topic next to the number, find it in chapter seven and jump on the internet to look up the paper - some of the papers will be written in a more academic style than this book, but will contain far more specifics if you are after them.

I dish out a few tips and tricks for when it comes to improving sleep - please look at these as tips, and not rules because by-in-large I have most definitely ignored all my own advice in the process of writing this. So know that perfect sleep does not require perfection but better sleep is possible with a little purpose in our efforts. I hope you enjoy what I have to offer - and if you are already dying to get the tips and tools, and you are happy to skip the biology lesson, feel free to jump to chapter six.

Chapter One - What is Sleep?

They say that sleep is the cousin of death, this could just be poetic and I have no idea where this leaves wakefulness in the family tree but I assume the metaphor is more often used to describe the similarity between the state of being unconscious during sleep and being unconscious after death. Aside from looking very similar, sleep and death also share a great deal of mystery - even in the academic realm. It may come as a shock to learn how little we actually know about this thing that most of us are doing every night. Scientists have been studying sleep for many years, and we have a good understanding of the different stages of sleep, the importance of sleep for physical and mental health, and the effects of sleep disorders.

For a very long time it was just assumed that when we close our eyes at the end of the day it was because our brains had just run out of juice and needed time to shut down, reboot, and restart. Intuitively this makes sense, if you have ever had a remote control toy run out of battery and grind to halt its almost like it needs a nap in the charger before it can be played with again. From the outside our bodies look like they do a very similar thing. Slowing of the limbs, a blunted sense of humour, and heavy eyelids, which can all be reversed with a little sleep, However, with the progress made in neuroscience and our ability to see what going on in the inside of our brain we now have a very different view on what is going on in there. We know that the brain goes through five different stages of activity during sleep. The first four stages are called stage 1, 2, 3, and 4; with 4 being the deepest stage, the fifth stage is called rapid eye movement (REM) sleep; where dreams are had and where our eyes move rapidly (2). But probably what is most apparent about sleep is that the scientists that research it are not the most creative when it comes to naming things.

Every time you fall asleep you start a cyclic pattern of moving through all five stages of sleep, the duration of which varies from person to person but on average it takes about 90 minutes to complete the cycle (3). By using neuroimaging techniques scientists have been able to watch the brain while it sleeps and they have found that not all cycles are the same throughout the night. It appears that during the first half of the night we spend more time in the first four stages of sleep, getting progressively deeper with each cycle. In the second half of the night we spend more dreaming in REM sleep, this is perhaps why it is easier to recall dreams when our alarms disrupt us while in this state (4). Below I have put together a mock chart visual representation of what a night's sleep could look like:

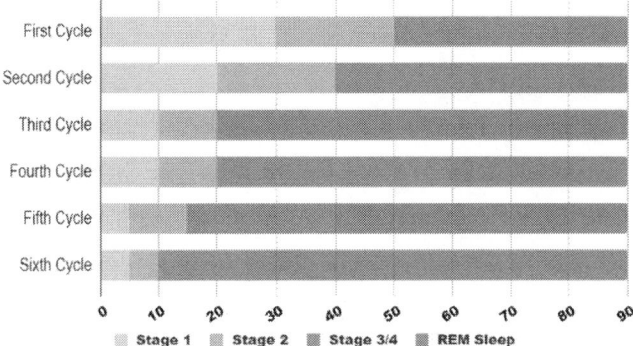

So why do we have all of these different kinds of sleep? Short answer is we don't know yet, but broadly speaking we know that REM and Non-REM sleep have differing effects on our body.

Non-REM sleep plays a crucial role in maintaining the body's physical health. During Non-REM sleep, the body goes into "repair mode" and takes the opportunity to perform essential maintenance tasks such as muscle repair, tissue growth, and hormone regulation. The body also works to strengthen the immune system, which is why you might feel lethargic and sleepy when you are under the weather in an attempt to bolster recovery. One of the most significant benefits of deep sleep is its ability to promote the release of growth hormone, which is essential for tissue repair and muscle growth. This is particularly beneficial for people who engage in regular physical activity, as it helps to repair and rebuild muscle tissue that has been damaged during exercise. Deep sleep also plays a crucial role in regulating glucose metabolism, which is why it has been linked to the prevention of obesity and diabetes. Studies have shown that individuals who experience poor sleep or have sleep disorders such as insomnia have an increased risk of developing obesity and diabetes. Additionally, deep sleep has been linked to a reduction in the risk of heart disease. Research has shown that individuals who experience poor sleep or have sleep disorders such as sleep apnoea have an increased risk of developing hypertension and cardiovascular disease. This is thought to be due to the impact of poor sleep on the regulation of blood pressure and heart rate.

Not that we need all of the doom and gloom to motivate us to go to bed, but it would feel a miss if I forgot to mention how good it is for you to hit the hay on occasion. There will be more on the specifics later on in chapters four and five.

Since Non-REM is more concerned with the physical rejuvenation of the body, you should expect that REM sleep is mostly beneficial for mental health and primarily emotional regulation. One of the most well-established benefits of REM sleep is its ability to consolidate and process emotional memories. Research has shown that during REM sleep, the brain replays and organizes emotional experiences that were encountered during the day. This process helps to integrate the emotional information into long-term memory, which can aid in emotional regulation and the ability to cope with stress. Additionally, REM sleep has been found to play a crucial role in regulating emotional responses. Studies have shown that individuals who experience poor REM sleep or have sleep disorders such as insomnia, have an increased risk of developing emotional disorders such as depression and anxiety. This is thought to be due to the impact of poor REM sleep on the regulation of emotional responses. Furthermore, REM sleep has been found to be associated with emotional regulation through the process of dreaming. During REM sleep, the brain generates vivid and often emotionally charged dreams, which can serve as a form of emotional self-regulation. Dreams may serve as a way to process and make sense of unresolved emotional conflicts, which can promote emotional well-being. One way I like to conceptualize REM sleep is as if our brains are running a "life-simulator" - like a pilot would have a flight simulator, and in this simulator it conjures up old experiences or predicts new ones to safely test whether or not all the emotion response buttons are working efficiently. Just in case you are not practicing your "how you doing's" enough in the mirror, your brain will do it for you while you sleep. Unfortunately sometimes our brains are less concerned with how 'cool' you look around your crush and are more interested in keeping you alive during life threatening event and so every now and then it may simulate some hand to hand combat, or running away from a monster while wearing flippers on you feet - I don't know, dreams are weird.

What I find to be super interesting about these two types of sleep is how well they have worked together in keeping our species (and others) running so smoothly for so long, and how it can adapt to fit our body's needs. If a person has been pushing their body hard in the gym, the brain will prioritize deep sleep over REM, and vice versa if the day has been particularly emotionally taxing and a little extra REM sleep would be helpful to process the feelings. There are limitations however, our brains will always put deep sleep cycles first so running short on REM cycles can be common if we have low sleep volume and since 60+% of our REM sleep happens in the later cycles, setting that alarm 2 hours early can have a disproportionately large toll on our emotional health. There are also a handful of lifestyle factors that disrupt our sleep; we will hear about these later on, but for one reason or another, things can tend to fall apart in some very peculiar ways.

So to answer the Question, What is Sleep? I guess we can say it is a mysterious yet necessary biological occurrence that helps keep our systems running smoothly.

Chapter Two - Sleep and the Brain

So now we know a little more about what sleep is and the differing stages, the next topic we should cover is how all this happens - what exactly puts us to sleep, and if you're not interested in physiology at all you should still read this chapter for the hands-on experience of being bored to sleep. The Process of falling sleep is a complex process that involves the coordination of various neural pathways in the brain. The main neural pathways involved in the regulation of sleep include the suprachiasmatic nucleus (SCN) of the hypothalamus, the ventrolateral preoptic area (VLPO) of the hypothalamus, and the ascending arousal system. Don't worry if this is all jargon, the names will not be in the final exam but being able to recall them later will take your dinner party banter to the next level.

Let's start with the suprachiasmatic nucleus; the 'soup-ra-kai-as-matic' nucleus is located in the hypothalamus and is considered the primary pacemaker of the sleep-wake cycle. I like to think of it as the super charismatic nucleus because of how well he can convince us of the time, plus if you say it fast no one can tell the difference. The SCN receives input from the retina and is responsible for regulating the circadian rhythm, which is the 24-hour sleep-wake cycle. At a cellular level, the SCN consists of a network of neurons that are responsible for maintaining the circadian rhythm. These neurons express various clock genes, such as BMAL1, and PER2, which work in a ebb and flow routine that completes a loop about every 24 hours. The SCN also receives input from the eyes, which provides information about the light-dark cycle. When light comes in it activates a protein called Melanopsin which promotes the production of Melatonin (which is also what your GP may prescribe you if you struggle with sleep) (5).

So now we know about the internal clock, let's look at what actually puts us down and gets us up. The ventrolateral preoptic area (VLPO) is also located in the hypothalamus and plays a role in promoting sleep. The VLPO sends inhibitory signals to the ascending arousal system, which helps to decrease wakefulness and promote sleep. Over the course of the day this region (and a few others) accumulate a neurotransmitter called Adenosine. Adenosine is the "A" in ATP - which is our body's version of fuel, and what our metabolism works so hard to turn food into. The VLPO measures the levels of Adenosine to gauge

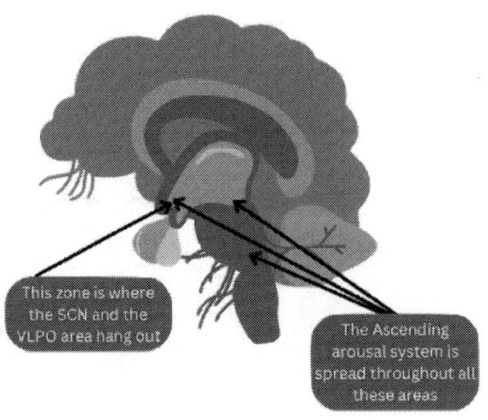

how much wakefulness we have had, and once we reach a tipping point it starts preparing us for sleep. You can think of this area as the "debbie-downer" that tells the Ascending Arousal System to quiet down once it's had enough. This mechanism may come up again later because when it gets out of balance it tends to have negative impacts on our ability to have quality deep sleep (6,7).

The ascending arousal system is a network of neurons that originate in the brainstem and travel through the hypothalamus, and the cerebral cortex. This system promotes wakefulness and arousal and is active during the day. The ascending arousal system is composed of several neurotransmitters and neuromodulators, including dopamine, norepinephrine, and histamine. Dopamine being a major player here as it involves many functions in the brain including motivation levels, physical movement, emotion regulation, and reward pathways. There are lifestyle factors here and agonist drugs that will come back up in later chapters that can lead to dysregulated dopamine levels and so to imbalances in arousal and issues with sleep. Norepinephrine; or nor-adrenaline you may know it as, and Histamines you might recognise and being involved with our stress response. It goes without saying that in most cases it is beneficial to be awake and alert during periods of stress which makes sense that this system is put into action when stress is present - be it from a thrilling event or something like pollen. The balance between the activity of the ascending arousal system and the VLPO is crucial for the regulation of sleep (8). There are a few other regions of importance but for brevity's sake know that we have a light controlled biological clock, a "hype you up" system, and a "you have done enough" system that govern our sleep by and large.

Now if you going to look at a brain and find these areas you may be surprised to know how small they all are, and this is because our brains do far more than turn us on and off - I would go as far as to say that it's most important function is to generate cognitive awareness (to be you), however sleep is very important to do this efficiently. The relationship between sleep and cognition is complex and bidirectional, with sleep affecting cognitive performance and cognitive performance affecting sleep. Studies have shown that a lack of sleep can lead to a decline in cognitive performance, including attention, memory, and decision making (9). For example, lack of sleep can impair attention, making it difficult to focus on a task and maintain attention for an extended period. Memory can also be affected, leading to poor recall and retention of information. Executive functions, such as decision making and problem-solving, can also be impaired by a lack of sleep.

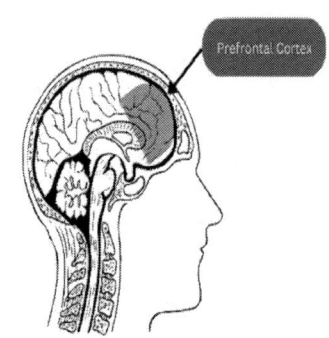

One area of the brain most affected by sleep deprivation is the prefrontal cortex which sits right up the front of the skull behind your forehead. This part of the brain is responsible for all of our higher order thinking and goal directed planning. It's what helps us problem solve to achieve a goal, stops us from being antisocial and punching people who cut in line at the supermarket, and also helps us with spatial awareness - its the part that only finishes developing after adolescence, to give you an idea of how you may act when its not fully online. This is why staying up all night building flat-pack furniture with your roommates is not often advised - especially if you like your roommates.

    The effects of sleep deprivation on cognitive performance are not only short-term but also long-term. Chronic sleep deprivation can lead to long-lasting cognitive impairment, including memory decline and a decline in overall cognitive function; think Alzheimer's or Dementia at the extreme end (10). This is particularly concerning in populations that are at risk for sleep deprivation, such as shift workers and individuals with sleep disorders. In contrast, sufficient and good quality sleep can enhance cognitive performance, including attention, memory, and executive function. This is the definition of waking up on the right side of the bed.

Chapter Three - Hormones and Sleep

As with every process in our bodies hormones play a significant role, unlike neural events in the Brian hormones tend to have longer duration of effect and require larger (all body) systems to coordinate properly to work well. In this chapter I will go over three of the main ones - in my opinion, and again if physiology is not your thing try your best to stay with me here I will do my best to spice up some of the intricacies of "bore"mones.

The first one I will cover we have already touched on, Melatonin, it comes from the pineal gland once the super charismatic nucleus stops receiving light, remember? A large portion of it also comes from the gut and it goes to work all over our body, even in our bones promoting relaxation and turning down any arousal we might have. One of the major ingredients we need to make melatonin is called tryptophan "trip-toe-fan", which is a super fun protein name to say in comparison to others. Tryptophan is also a major ingredient in making serotonin which is key to our "feel good response", so plenty of reasons to keep up our protein consumption. Foods that are high in tryptophan include turkey, chicken, eggs, cheese, yogurt, soybeans, and pumpkin seeds. However, it is important to note that the relationship between tryptophan and melatonin is complex and not fully understood. The amount of tryptophan found in food may not always be enough to have an effect on melatonin production. Additionally, other factors such as stress and exposure to light can tend to affect melatonin production more than tryptophan levels alone. It's also important to note that taking pure tryptophan supplements is not recommended without seeking advice from a healthcare provider first, although some of the more recent evidence is promising (11) - no guarantees though, sometimes it can just go straight through you. On occasion melatonin therapy can be used for people with sleeping issues but the evidence for it actually having a positive effect is poor or mainly a placebo effect at best (12). One reason for this is as you increase the amount of a hormone in the system, the less the body wants to listen to it - kind of like how parents get numb to the sounds of their own kids yelling and screaming and stop responding, our brains get better and tuning out the melatonin screaming in its receptors. However, sometimes taking a pill can put you at ease knowing you are doing something, and being at ease is great if you are trying to sleep.

    Natural Melatonin production follows very closely to our biological clock, it peaks when it becomes dark and stays pretty high throughout the night. Artificial lighting is really the biggest issue that disrupts this process, because even if the sun goes down our brains have a tough time telling the difference while we still have light coming in our eyes. Levels only begin to drop once the VLPO (from before) has cleared enough adenosine for the arousal system to kick back into action. This is also a time sensitive process as the VLPO learns how fast it needs to work at, this is why having an ever changing bedtime/alarm clock can leave you waking up groggy and still full of adenosine. Age also plays a role. It's a tough point to prove and it might just be correlation, but the older we get the less melatonin we tend to produce, the smaller our VLPO areas gets, as well as a few other fairly important hormones too - meaning we get worse at recovering the older the machine gets.

The opposition to melatonin's sleep promoting effects come from a super group cluster of hormones called the Catecholamines (honestly the pronunciation of this varies all over the world but I will give you this one "Cat-a-cole-la-means".) This group includes Adrenaline, nor-adrenaline, dopamine, and not technically but practically Cortisol too. When I talk about "the stress response" this is a crew I am referring to, and they launch into action every time you have to. Sometimes they are so effective at launching into action they even do it when you "think" you might have too - imagine quickly that there is an angry dog foaming at the mouth across the room from you - you just had a little spurt of catecholamines from your adrenal glands.

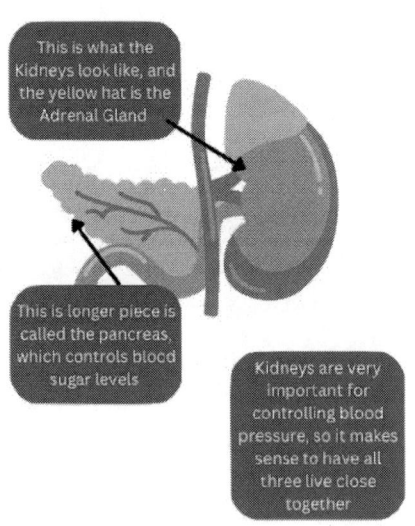

This group of hormones are great at turning on the ascending arousal system in the brain, but they also have effects like increased blood pressure, heart rate, and blood sugar levels.

Which are all great things to help you stay awake alert and ready for action, it's only when we become chronically stressed - like when we have a person in our lives that's a little unpleasant to be around, or a 30 year mortgage over our heads, or excessive vigorous exercise, or chronic pain etc. etc., that it can impact our sleep in a negative way. There are also some medications that can cause issues with this balance also such as, Duromine (a weight loss pill), Corticosteroid injections, as well as drugs like Caffeine and Nicotine/Amphetamines. These compounds all increase the amount of Catecholamines in our bodies and in the long term reduce your sleep quality, and even lead to things like insomnia.

It's not only stress that swings the tides of Catecholamines though, there is a natural rhythm that ebbs and flows over the 24 hour cycle. Levels will automatically peak right before you wake up, the arousal system feels this peaks and arouses you. This is why some of us struggle to sleep in on our days off, we don't have the ability to control these levels very well. On the plus side, having a strong regular peak time can help you from feeling groggy during the week, and the more often you wake up at the same time the more ingrained the rhythm becomes. One interesting note though about how we can have some outside influence on this is that if you have a "big event" on the next day, or you are sleeping in a new environment, or maybe you have a job where you are "on call" during the night, there will actually be a smaller spike in the morning. Downside to this is thought that your stress hormones levels are elevated all night and your levels of deep sleep and REM sleep will be trash - makes you feel for all the new parents and call-out workers out there (13). We also in general will get a peak of these whenever we are awake and in the dark, two-fold if you are puffed, awake and in the dark. The reason for this is very obvious if we look at it from a historical view; how often before the invention of lights, do you think our species went night running for reasons that did not involve running for our lives - very rarely, and so stress responses are very linked to that kind of activity.

    The last one I will touch on is growth hormone (GH), not that it controls sleep to a large degree but it is interesting and very beneficial for your health. During sleep, GH is released in pulses, with the highest levels of GH release occurring during deep sleep (stage 3/4). The release of GH during deep sleep is thought to promote physical recovery and repair of the body, this is why it is also called "the fountain of youth" hormone. GH has anabolic effects on the body, helping to build and repair tissues, bones, and muscles. Studies have shown that people with insomnia have lower levels of GH compared to people who sleep normally. Low levels of GH are also associated with poor physical recovery and repair, which can contribute to a host of other health problems, such as decreased muscle mass, increased body fat, decreased bone density, and an increased risk of injury.

    GH is sometimes prescribed by doctors but mainly for the treatment of pituitary dwarfism, not for sleep issues. In the world of sports however, the use of GH is sometimes used to help with sport performance and muscle gain - which it is very effective for however not recommended, as taking excess GH can have very negative side effects, including joint pain, carpal tunnel syndrome, and an increased risk of diabetes and cancer, also it can cause an imbalance of other hormones in the body. So, although GH can be very beneficial for our health, it is best to try and maximize your natural levels by getting enough deep sleep and keeping your catecholamines low. Taking extra GH will not help your sleep and can lead to worse health outcomes - which is unfortunate because taking a pill would be much easier.

All up it is good to have the perspective that sleep, and especially good sleep is not just an on/off switch. It involves fast mechanical parts of the brain, yes, but the fuel and instructions for those parts are much slower moving hormones which can be thrown out of balance in a variety of weird and wonderful ways.

Chapter Four - Sleep and Physical Health

There is a saying that goes something like "you can't out-exercise a bad diet", I'm not sure who said it first but it's on the internet so it must be true. I would like to start this chapter by going one step further and claim "you can't out-diet a bad sleep".

Here is a neat pyramid diagram showing the sequence of importance when it comes to progressive health - basically the rule to follow is, you can't get the

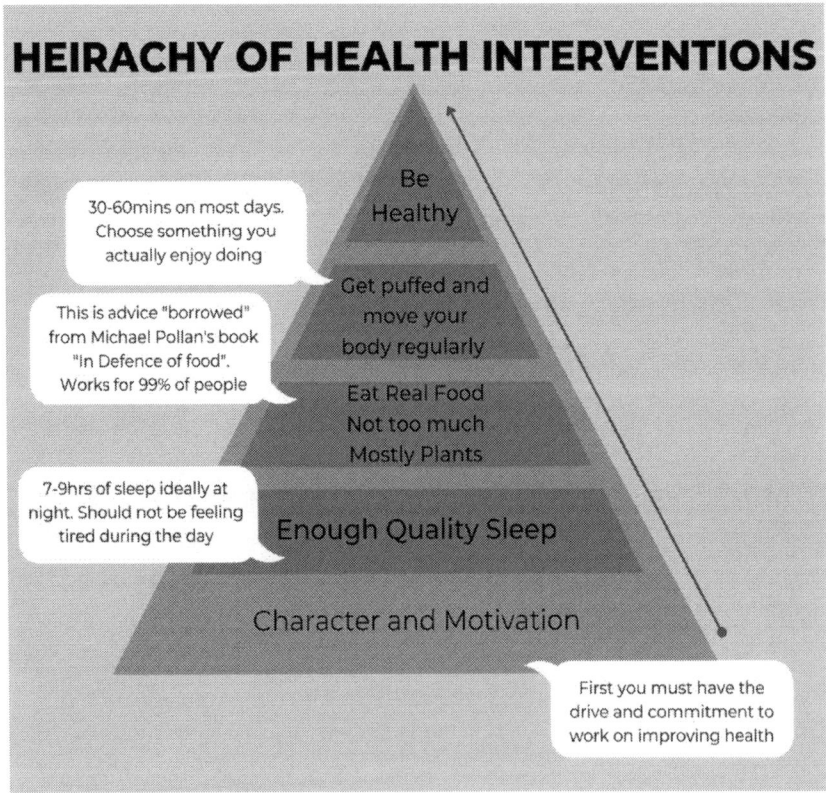

most from one level until the level below it has been achieved.

So you can tell how highly I rate sleep as being the foundation to health, in this chapter I will cover some of the well-known and not so well known ways it makes a direct impact on our physical bodies.

Let's start with metabolic health, which is just things that concern how we get and use energy in our body as well as things like cholesterol, blood sugar, and fat storage. Sleep plays a crucial role in regulating appetite, and disruptions to sleep can lead to an increased appetite, particularly for high-calorie foods. Studies have shown that people who get insufficient sleep tend to eat more and have a higher body mass index (BMI) than people who get enough sleep (14). Sleep plays a role in balancing hormones that control appetite and energy balance, such as ghrelin and leptin. Ghrelin is a hormone that increases appetite, kicks starts cravings for sweet carb based foods, and makes us want to sit around more often digesting the foods. Getting less sleep increases your levels of this hormone plus, gives you more time to fill that appetite with food (15).

Just to add fuel to the fire, remember how broken sleep spiked the stress hormones? Cortisol in particular is great at helping us store fat for emergencies and at keeping our cholesterol and blood sugar high - just in case we need to run from something. However, if we don't need to be running all that extra fat and sugar in our blood can lead to things like high blood pressure (as there is more gunk to pump around), increased body fat (specifically belly fat), atherosclerosis (fatty build-up's in our arteries) and insulin resistance (diabetes). Hang on there is more, Insulin resistance itself also kicks start cravings for high carb foods as well, in an attempt to trigger more insulin to be released. It really is a series of unfortunate events that keep piling up, all due to a little lost sleep (16).

Before we even get the foods into us though, being well rested is great for making mindful decisions about food choices, and better decisions in general too. Sleep affects the activity of the reward centre in the brain. Studies have shown that sleep deprivation can lead to an increase in the activity of the reward centre, which can make really sweet and fatty foods doubly rewarding to us, making us want them even more (17). This is why after a long night of partying with your friends, a deep fried feed will seem like the best meal of earth. Triggering the reward system and making you feel far less second hand - it's not exactly that hot chips are a magic cure, but they can trick your brain into feeling better about its situation.

Long term disrupted sleep, and chronically going through these patterns in most cases will lead to obesity. Having extra padding may not actually affect your health or sleep to a large degree, but there is a turning point where it can become an issue. I won't go over all the ways obesity can be an issue - it would take too long, and I feel that most humans nowadays have had it beat into them so hard through the news and media that I don't have to double down on it. One I will touch one is how excess body/belly/central fat can lead to things like sleep apnoea.

This is where sleep is disrupted or "shallowed" by our bodies not being able to breathe while we are asleep. There are a handful of way this happens (hormones etc.,) but for me the most obvious one is because our lungs begin to struggle under the weight of our bodies (18). It is quite literally sleeping with a weight on your chest. It's a really nasty condition because unless our bed buddies tell us it's happening we may never know. We can just wake up feeling unrested, unaware our bodies have been wrestling to breathe all night. Treatment can involve wearing a mask and an air tank at night, which can make sleep feel a little less comfortable can do wonders for sleep quality and afford you more sleep hours to help with weight loss.

    The second most common health effects from sleep could be on the gastrointestinal system - the internal tube that starts at your lips and ends at your "end". There are two areas of this system that are more affected than others when it comes to sleep, I will start with the top end. You may have heard of GERD (or GORD depending where you are from), it is a condition that occurs when stomach acid flows back into the esophagus, causing damage to the esophageal lining. GERD can range in severity from mild to severe. Mild GERD is characterized by occasional symptoms, such as heartburn, spicy burps, and acid regurgitation. More severe GERD, is characterized by more frequent and severe symptoms, such as heartburn, acid regurgitation, chest pain, and difficulty swallowing. These symptoms may occur at any time and can be persistent, interfering with daily activities and quality of life. The relationship between sleep and GERD is bidirectional, good quality deep sleep helps normalize the amount of stomach acid you produce - reducing the severity of the symptoms (19). The other way though, GERD most commonly affects people if they eat their last meal right before they lay down - or if the meal was quite large, which in turn makes getting enough deep sleep very hard. Using things like over the counter antacids or stronger prescription drugs can help break the cycle and help get that sleep back, although long term use of either of these methods tends to do more harm than good. It can slow protein digestion - which we need to make melatonin, and it reduces how well we absorb some of the B vitamins - which promote health and energy levels (20).

The second area of the gastrointestinal system that needs good sleep to maintain is the bowels. Where we absorb all the nutrients from food and turn it into poop. Moving food through the bowels actually takes a lot of smooth muscle coordination, this is all out of our conscious control and relies more on hormone balance to move at the correct speed so we don't end up all blocked up, or with too much liquid in the mix. Deep sleep helps maintain a good level of these hormones and keeps your bowel movements consistent - in texture and frequency. Too

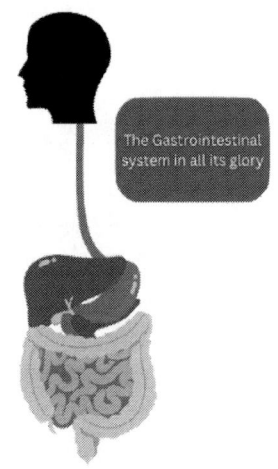

The Gastrointestinal system in all its glory

little deep sleep can leave you in a rush, squirting, and/or hurting. Which are all things I assume we want to avoid while on the loo. Studies show that people with poor sleep habits are more likely to develop conditions like irritable bowel syndrome (IBS) (21).

    IBS is an umbrella name that covers a heap of very similar feeling conditions such as, ulcerative colitis, crohn's disease, leaky gut syndrome, and even some allergies can fall in here too. This is a large topic so I do my best to only skim over the basics. Remember how I was saying before about how our bodies often read lack of sleep as a reason to turn on the stress response? Well when our bowels are stressed out our internal gut security system goes on high alert looking for suspicious characters that may be causing the stress. You can imagine them an intestine police if that helps - but instead of handcuffs and prison they work more like suicide bombers and destroy invaders on the spot, causing a lot of inflammation. When these guys are on high alert they tend to become suspicious of everything, including the walls of your intestine - this is called an autoimmune reaction. Funny enough, having the suicide bomber police force attacking the inside your bowels can actually irritate the bowel itself, which can lead to pain, bloating, and very urgent, liquidy stools (poops). I say this in a light hearted way but for people living with IBS it is a very serious and uncomfortable condition - it can really impact quality of life for these people. As much as I promote sleep as being great, it can only be used to help reduce the stress response in these conditions. So although it cannot cure IBS, it should be one factor to keep in mind during treatment of these conditions.

Just to play the devil's advocate here I will propose

a theory to you. What if we miss enough sleep and stay on

alert so long that we tire our immune system out and it

stops causing things like IBS? In theory yes this can work,

however having a depressed immune system can actually

have its own negative side effects. A chronically depressed

immune response, also known as immunodeficiency, is a

condition in which the body's immune system is not able to effectively fight off infections, illnesses, and diseases. This can lead to a variety of signs and symptoms that can

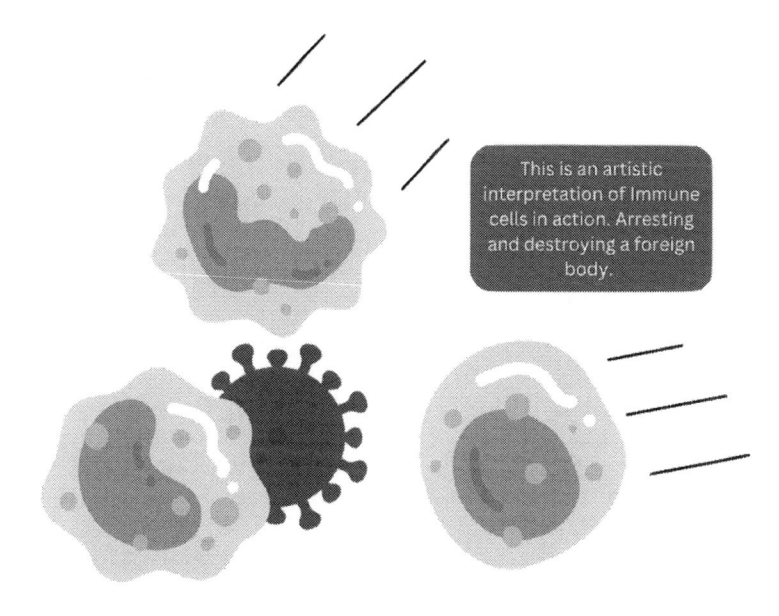

This is an artistic interpretation of Immune cells in action. Arresting and destroying a foreign body.

affect a person's overall health and quality of life. People with a chronically depressed immune response may experience frequent infections, such as colds, flu, and pneumonia, which may also have more severe symptoms. Additionally, wounds and injuries may take longer to heal and they may be more susceptible to infections in the wound. It can also make a person more susceptible to autoimmune disorders, such as rheumatoid arthritis, lupus, and multiple sclerosis. Furthermore, people with a chronically depressed immune response may have an increased risk of developing certain types of cancer, such as lymphomas and leukaemia's. Allergies and asthma may also be more prevalent (22). So although I applaud the out-of-box thinking, this theory is firmly debunked.

As we can see there are many aspects of physical health that rely on sleep to function properly (and many more I have left off the list here too). Sleep, particularly deep sleep, is a great way to give our bodies time to check on the warning lights that have popped up on our metaphorical dashboards. It's less like parking your car up for the night and more like checking your car in for a service - except it's free, and the mechanic working on it has amazing google reviews and has been doing it since the dawn of our species.

Chapter Five - Sleep and Mental Health

Tigger warning: Suicide and Self Harm.

The relationship between sleep and mental health is equally complex to that of physical health and shares many similarities. In this chapter I will cover similar topics but with more of a focus on how it can affect our mental wellbeing. Sleep disturbances can contribute to the development of mental health conditions such as depression, anxiety, and post-traumatic stress disorder (PTSD), and conversely, mental health conditions can lead to sleep disturbances. I will touch on some of the more common ways this appears in real life as well as the potential protective effects of good sleep.

A lot of the starting blocks for mental health actually begin with the physical body, so although this may feel like a step back it will come full circle soon enough. Depression is a mental health condition characterized by persistent feelings of sadness, hopelessness, and a loss of interest in activities. It is believed to be caused by imbalances in certain neurotransmitters, including serotonin, in the brain. Anxiety disorders - Like PTSD, form a category of mental health diagnoses, and are treated through therapy and medication. Serotonin also plays a role in regulating anxiety levels, and low levels of serotonin have been linked to anxiety disorders. Even though the one neurotransmitter is involved with both conditions, these two can occur separately or together. What causes this is often due to other factors like genetics or life experience. One type of medications that are used to treat these conditions are called selective serotonin reuptake inhibitors (SSRI's), which work in the brain to increase the amount of free serotonin floating between brain cells. These SSRI's are fairly common prescriptions worldwide and can have some great results - they can also be hit and miss at times too, so not a perfect cure (23). One thing to note though is how important having regular balanced levels of serotonin must be for our mental health.

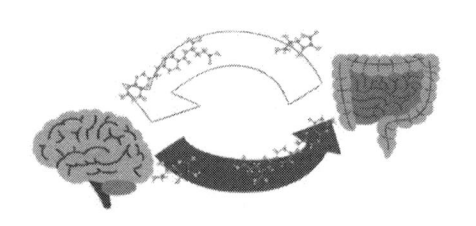

    An area of recent findings that has gained interest in this field is the concept of the gut-brain axis - how the brain affects the gut and even how the gut affects the brain. It is estimated that around 90% of the body's serotonin is produced in the gut, with the remaining 10% produced in the brain (24). While the majority of serotonin is produced and stored in the enterochromaffin cells located throughout the gut, it is also produced by other cells in the gut such as the enteric neurons and immune cells. The process of making serotonin in the gut starts with the protein tryptophan - remember this guy? As well as making melatonin, he also plays a role in making serotonin too - very handy. Although, like we read in the last chapter, our gastrointestinal tract works best when we are well rested and so, a lack of sleep can disrupt how well we are digesting proteins and producing these important chemicals. It is important to note that the gut-brain axis is a two-way street, as the gut also receives signals from the brain, which can affect the production of serotonin and other neurotransmitters. This highlights the intricate and complex relationship between the gut and the brain and how they work together to regulate our mental well-being.

    The next one we will look at will be some of the cognitive effects on our mental health. Temporal discounting refers to the phenomenon in which the perceived value of a reward decreases as the delay to receive it increases. In other words, people tend to prefer smaller rewards that are available sooner over larger rewards that are available later. This phenomenon has been extensively studied in the field of psychology and economics and has been shown to play a role in decision-making, impulse control, and addiction. Temporal discounting is thought to be influenced by a number of factors, including differences in impulsivity, delay aversion, and sensitivity to reward - which are all behaviours that become more common the less we sleep (25,26). So in the same way that the fast food feed becomes more appealing after a long night out, so can many other things including high risk behaviour. Top of the list for risky temptations is that of suicide ideation, and self-harm. Sleep disturbances, such as insomnia and nightmares, have been consistently linked to an increased risk of suicide. Studies have shown that individuals with insomnia are at a higher risk of suicidal ideation and suicide attempts compared to those without insomnia. Similarly, individuals with nightmares have been found to have a higher risk of suicide attempts, particularly in those with post-traumatic stress disorder (PTSD). Insomnia, in particular, has been found to be a significant predictor of suicide risk, even after controlling for other risk factors such as depression and anxiety. This may be due to the fact that insomnia can exacerbate feelings of hopelessness and helplessness, and may make it more difficult for individuals to cope with negative emotions (27).

Along these same lines of thinking, there is a growing body of research that suggests a link between sleep disturbances and addictive behaviours. Studies have shown that individuals with insomnia or other sleep disturbances are more likely to engage in addictive behaviours, such as substance abuse, gambling, and Internet addiction (28,29). One theory is that sleep deprivation can disrupt the balance of neurotransmitters in the brain, such as dopamine, which plays a key role in reward-seeking behaviours. When dopamine levels are disrupted, an individual may seek out other sources of pleasure or reward, such as drugs or gambling, to compensate for the lack of dopamine. Additionally, sleep deprivation can lead to increased stress and anxiety, which can make it more difficult for individuals to cope with negative emotions. This may make them more vulnerable to engaging in addictive behaviours as a means of self-medication. One aspect of this that I find very interesting is that most; if not all, of our commonly addictive behaviours are sleep agonists - they actively reduce the quality and our ability to sleep, I will cover a few here. Number one on this list (in terms of commonness, not impact) is internet addiction. This covers a range of web surfing from shopping, online gaming/gambling, porn, and worst of the worst - social media. These kinds of self-soothing addictive behaviours affect sleep in two major ways, the first is the obvious light pollution into the suprachiasmatic nucleus. This tricks the brain into thinking the sun is still up and slows melatonin production. Using a "blue-light filter" can help but is not perfect or a justification for playing fortnite till 2am (fortnite is an online shooting game, for those of us out-of-the-know). Secondly, the big reason why these behaviours are addictive in the first place is because they get our dopamine flowing, which helps fuel the ascending arousal system and keeps us alert. These online activities are designed to keep us engaged by using the "what if" factor, and every time your brain thinks "what if" you get a little hit of dopamine - what if this next bet pays off, what if this next video is funny, what if someone likes my post etc. etc. We all know the feeling, it's why the infinite scroll is so hard to put down (30).

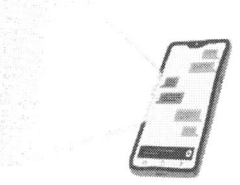

    Substance addictions are another kettle of fish, there are some that increase the catecholamines (stress response hormones) like nicotine, amphetamines, and caffeine. Even if you feel like these don't have an effect on you, or in some cases people even find them relaxing, this is more of a subjective feeling and doesn't override the chemistry going on in your brain. One theory of why these chemicals can have a soothing effect is that the boost in catecholamines works as an answer to why we are not feeling well. In other words, our brains are saying "hmm something feels off but I don't know what..." so we bump up the dopamine and the nor-adrenaline and then the brain says "ahhh thats it, I'm stressed, that's why I feel off now I can relax knowing I am appropriately responding to the world". Caffeine also has a dual effect because when it enters the brain, it blocks the adenosine receptors in the VLPO. Remember from chapter three, where we covered that measuring the adenosine levels is how the VLPO tracks how tired you should feel? When these receptors are blocked it's like putting a blindfold on the VLPO, and he has no idea until you are able to break down the caffeine molecules - which on average takes about 3-6 hours (31). Now I know (more than I would like to admit) how handy this can be if you are trying to ignore how tired you are, but a 3-6 hour delay is probably something I would complain about if it happened to me in an airport - so just be grateful the VLPO can't run screaming to the front desk, and do your best to keep flights on time.

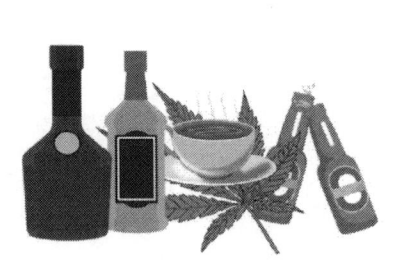

    Alcohol and Marijuana are another pair of substances that affect sleep. Although not commonly thought of as "addictive-addictive", they are used regularly for self-soothing and sometimes even thought to help with sleep. In both cases their most detrimental effect is on REM sleep. Alcohol and tetrahydrocannabinol (THC), the main psychoactive compound found in Marijuana have been shown to increase the amount of time spent in REM sleep but only during the first half of the night, and to decrease the amount of time spent in REM sleep during the second half of the night. This leads to a reduction of overall REM sleep time, which we know is the most important stage of sleep for emotional processing. As expected, long-term use of alcohol and THC can lead to chronically low REM sleep levels and to increased levels of emotional distress; like depression and anxiety. It can seem like a self-perpetuating cycle e.g. more distress equals more soothing equals less REM equals more distress and so on (32,33). Cannabidiol (CBD), on the other hand, is the non-psychoactive compound found in Marijuana. It has been shown to have therapeutic potential for a variety of conditions, including sleep disorders. The exact mechanism by which CBD improves sleep is not fully understood. It has been shown to reduce stress and work against the dopamine and catecholamines, it also has effects on the suprachiasmatic nucleus; convincing it that it's time to wind down and relax, but the exact mechanisms are still unknown and more research is probably needed before I go launching recommendations like that.

 It's good to be mindful of how closely sleep disturbances are associated with an increase in risky, and sometimes self-destructive behaviour. Also, how temporal discounting- the phenomenon where the perceived value of a reward decreases as the delay to receive it increases, influences decision-making, impulse control, and addiction. Additionally, we now know how lack of REM sleep can put into action that emotional regulation - self soothing cycle. It is clear that sleep plays a crucial role in maintaining mental well-being. Therefore, it really is something that healthcare professionals could be screening for in individuals who are at risk of suicide, mental health conditions and addictive behaviours.

Chapter Six - How to Improve Your Sleep
This is where the work begins

So we come to the final chapter, and this is the one where I will go over the practical things we can do to actually improve our sleep, and I will explain how to use the tool that makes up the second half of the book. If you were so desperate for help you skipped to this chapter, that's also fine. I wouldn't say there is anything ground breaking in the previous five, it's all fairly common sense but if something in this chapter refers back to earlier in the book it might be helpful to jump to that section to better understand the concept. The way I will structure this chapter will be different to the others. Basically I will go over the "sleep sheets" tool piece by piece and explain why I think these tools help and how to use them to their full potential. There are like seven tools on the sheet, and they are not in any order of effectiveness. Not everyone will find everyone helpful, and some may just seem impossible to fit into *your* life - but if we can understand the whys and how's of at least one of them, hopefully we can start moving in the right direction. As with most things in behaviour change activities - and there will be a bunch of health experts that will disagree with this but, it doesn't actually matter what you do, there are no hidden secrets or perfect plans, what matters is that find something you think will work, and you do that thing regularly, rain, hail, or snow.

Bed Times and Waking Times

First on the sheet we have a space to record the time we go to be, and the time we wake up. Bonus space has been added in case you want to do the math to see how many hours of sleep you are getting. The math is optional and less important but great to reflect back to if you want to track change or to measure if there is enough volume of sleep happening.
"Do I put this night's sleep hours or last nights?" great question, it's up to you, whatever works.

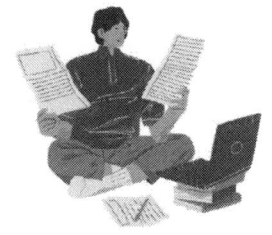

Why does this help? We know our sleep and wakefulness cycle runs on a 24 hour biological clock. This clock can be knocked out of sync with the real world for many reasons, but if we put effort into going to bed and waking up at similar times each day; even on weekends, we are able to recalibrate it. There is a little wiggle room here for some variance. The average person can shuffle their clock around by about 60 minutes without disrupting their hormone balances, so if you need a sleep in or a late night you have an hour. You shouldn't do both on the same night, but you can on the same day i.e. sleep in 30 mins, stay up 30 mins. Yes, real life can get in the way, and this is all perfect advice for perfect situations. If for some unforeseen yet certainly going to happen reason you blow out by 3 hours both ways that is fine, just know that if you do that for a week straight you will start to feel a little second hand. Another big "if" that might come up is if you start a new job, or you go overseas, or your routine changes and you need to switch your clock long term, this can be done. Ideally you would taper the changes over a week or so - little by little, for the easiest transition.

In the grand scheme of things, this might seem uber obvious. It's something that parents do with their kids because they know that tired kids are harder to handle - same rules apply to you, call it self-parenting. This is probably the easiest tool on the sheet, and a great first step if the other tools seem like a big commitment (34).

Bedtime Routine

This is another thing that's useful for parents in helping kids wind down for the day, sometimes we forget how we need to wind down too. On the sheet you will see a space to note the things you have done in the 60 mins leading up to going to bed. There are no rights or wrongs to put on this list - but you could say there are better or worse things though. One important thing to remember here is we are less interested in knowing what you do on any given day, this section is for tracking how consistent your routine is. Our brains really love routine and being able to guess what is going to happen next. When unpredictable things happen it costs our brain energy in order to stay agile and react to what's being thrown at it - and when the brain is spending energy when it doesn't want to it gets stressed out. As an example, if every night before bed we watched T.V, then did some stretches, then drank some water, then brushed our teeth and we did this every day for two weeks? Well on week three, by the time you are sipping your water the brain will be humming "ahh yes I know what's coming next, minty taste then a nap" and it can start shifting gears early to save on effort. A cool thing to note about routine setting that is if, by chance you cannot sleep for one reason or another, all you need to do is get up and repeat the process to give your brain a second chance at coordinating the sleep response (35).

    I will note a few things that live on the betterer side of activities to do in this 60 minute window. It's not a prescription because different lifestyles have different needs but let this be an inspiration if you are at a loss. Exposure to light is a key thing to track with all these pre-sleep activities, the brighter the light/the closer the light is to your face the harder it will be to slide into the first few stages of sleep. This puts "avoiding using technological devices" fairly high on the list 60 minutes leading up to bed time - maybe with the exception of old world technology, like an abacus if that's what you are into. Something that can help those first stages of sleep get into action is a shift in body temperature. As we reach stage 2 of the sleep cycle our body temp will begin to naturally drop as we get deeper and deeper into sleep - this is why sticking your foot out the side of the bed is so common. We can't exactly hack this process but doing something before bed that loosens our temperature settings can be helpful - like a hot shower. The more recently the gauge has had to readjust the easier it is to do it the second time as we fall asleep (36).

    The last one I will leave you with, that helps promote sleep is to engage in coitial activities (a bit of the, how's your father) if you catch my drift. This can be done solo or with a close friend completely up to you. Not only are there many social, spiritual, and physical health benefits to engaging in such activities it can also help people fall to sleep. During a mutually satisfactory bout of rumpy pumpy, both involved parties will activate a part of the nervous system called the sympathetic nervous system (which is sometimes called the fight or flight response), and then they will quickly shut it off after "completion". The shutting off part is the skill that's needed to help with promoting sleep, the smoother this transition is the easier it is for the first sleep cycle to begin (37,38). On this topic, while we have come this far I will note another handy tip. Remember how much our brain loves routine? This is true for spatial memory too, the room you are in and what you usually do in that room will help your brain predict what its next course of action should be. To help with sleep it pays to keep your bedroom as "sacred space", saved only for sleep and interpersonal physical relations. The more often you do other things in that room the harder it is for your brain to guess what is coming next i.e. if your bedroom is also your office or your home gym your brain might start gearing up to check emails or do burpees when it should be gearing down for sleep.

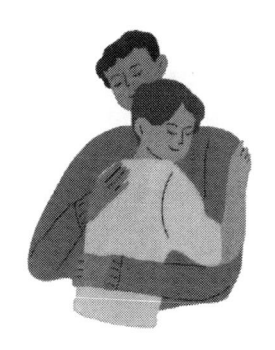

Must do's and Counting Wins

On the right side of the sheet you will see six spots to fill out titled "achievements" and "must do's". The first three are to be used to keep track and reflect on things you have done that day. This gives us space to note the things we are working on that we see as positive behaviours, no expectation to write things like "saved the world today" but writing things that we care about is the best use for this tool. In two months' time it can be very enlightening to see how habits change, grow, and develop - can also be used to keep ourselves accountable to our goals also. The act of reflecting on the day past is also a great cue to tell our brain that we have reached the end of the day, and to stop thinking of new tasks to do - gives it permission to sign off so to speak.

The must do's are fairly self-explanatory, these are things you must do tomorrow. Maybe finish a job you ran out of time on or a reminder to start a task for when you wake up. Our brains are freaking awesome at thinking about things, but they suck at holding onto thoughts. Jotting down thoughts is a great way to stop your brain juggling them all night - you can trust you won't forget them because paper is built to hold onto ideas, it just sucks at coming up with them (39). If there are more than three to do tomorrow you can pop them in the section below this one which I will cover next.

Brain Dump

This section is the largest tool of them all and probably requires the most amount of writing to do well. It really is a place to put any straggling thoughts you can't shake out, and it might take three or four shakes to get them all on paper and out of your head. You have the largest creative license on this tool and sometimes the more abstract the thoughts the better at getting you headspace in the right place (40).

A good analogy for why this is effective comes from that movie "Inception", that movie about entering other people's dreams and putting ideas in their heads - don't worry I don't think you have to watch it to understand it, but it might help, the movie is awfully long and drawn out. There is this one part though where Leonardo and Juno are sitting at a cafe and he is explaining how to control dreams. Then Juno realizes they are actually in a dream right now and the whole place starts to shake and fall apart because they are waking up. As far removed as the movie is from reality, this part has some credence. In order to keep the body sliding into dreamland it pays to forget the fact that you are trying to sleep. There is no faster way to become frustrated and to wake yourself up than to lie down and actively try to sleep - this is super common if you have an important thing to do the next day, and if that's the case just write it down in the brain dump and let your mind get back to drifting off. When we practice this skill it is called "stream of consciousness" because the ideas/words should flow like a stream without constraint or forceful guidance in any direction. Once we feel the "flow" of thoughts coming, pop the book down and let the mind continue to wander - anywhere except to the fact you are trying to sleep. This may take some skill and time to master. I have heard that using "story starters" as prompts can be helpful in the beginning.

Gratefulness Check

Back on the left side there is space to note one thing you are grateful for from this past day. Keeping a gratitude journal can be a simple yet effective way to improve your sleep. The act of writing down things that you are grateful for before going to bed can help to shift your focus away from negative thoughts and stressors, which can make it easier to fall asleep and stay asleep. Think of it as clearing the path from distracting weeds on the road to relaxation. Expressing gratitude has been shown to have a positive impact on mood and well-being, which can also contribute to better sleep. When you write down things that you are grateful for, you are focusing on the positive aspects of your life, which can help to counteract the negative thoughts and emotions that can keep you awake at night. Additionally, gratitude journaling can help to increase feelings of positivity and decrease symptoms of depression and anxiety, both of which can have a negative impact on sleep (41). One more benefit of gratitude journaling before sleep is that it can act as a form of mindfulness practice. Mindfulness is the ability to focus on the present moment without judgment, and it can be a helpful tool in managing insomnia and other sleep-related problems. By taking a few minutes to reflect on the things you are grateful for, you are training your mind to focus on the present and let go of any worries or stressors that may be keeping you awake.

Doodle Space

We are not all wordy people, I thought it would be great to have a space here for people who are more visual abstract thinkers. Drawing can potentially help with sleep by providing a form of relaxation and distraction from stressors or negative thoughts. The act of creating art can be therapeutic and can help to decrease feelings of anxiety or depression. It also allows people to release and express emotions that can be hard to put into words. Additionally, drawing can be a form of mindfulness practice, similar to gratitude journaling. Mindfulness is the ability to focus on the present moment without judgment, and it can be a helpful tool in managing insomnia and other sleep-related problems. By focusing on the act of drawing, you can distract your mind from any worries or stressors that may be keeping you awake.

It's important to note that drawing, like any other activity, should be done in moderation, especially close to bedtime. If you really - and I mean really, love drawing it may actually be too stimulating for the mind too close to bed can make it harder to fall asleep.

Sleep Hygiene Checks

This space here is to track and record any little tips this book, or anyone else have given you around sleep specifically. It could be avoiding the lights or having a small meal before bed etc., anything you go out of your way to do in order to help sleep happen. It might even be a place to track things like whether or not you have used a sleeping pill so you can see back measures if your use is increasing or decreasing.

We can visualize it as milking the most from every type of intervention. If knowing what to do is tier one, doing it is tier two, then tracking and reflecting on our habits is tier three and the best method to getting the most mileage from any one habit

Loving-Kindness

This tool is by far the "hippie-ist" one on the list but not without purpose. Loving-kindness, also known as "metta" in Buddhism, or "thoughts and prayers" in Judeo-

Christian religions, or "wishing the best" from a more secular point of view is a practice in which you cultivate a feeling of love and compassion for yourself and others. The goal of loving-kindness meditation is to develop a deep sense of warmth and compassion for oneself and others, and to increase one's ability to experience positive emotions such as joy, contentment, and love.

The practice of loving-kindness meditation typically involves sitting quietly and focusing on different people or groups of people, such as a loved one, a neutral person, a difficult person, or all beings. As you choose who you focus on each person or group, it's helpful to think of phrases such as "may you be happy, may you be healthy, may you be safe, may you be at ease." Or if this person is someone you know well, your thoughts may be more specific to their situation. Loving-kindness has been found to have a number of benefits for mental and emotional well-being. Research has shown that regular practice of loving-kindness meditation can lead to increased positive emotions, decreased negative emotions, and improved relationships with others. Loving-kindness meditation has been found to be effective in reducing symptoms of depression, anxiety, and stress. This is the main pathway that it can help with falling and staying asleep, it primes the body to feel well, relaxed and free from those arousing stress hormones (42).

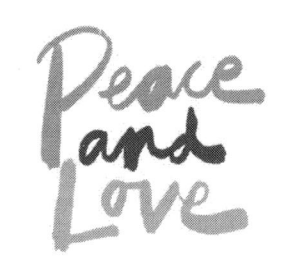

Today's Quotable

This is the last tool on the sheet, and the least sleep specific one. I have included this more as a way to reflect and track growth over time. The quote can come from anywhere or might just be an interesting thought you had that day. In the future when you look back these entries will serve as time capsules to show you what you felt was important at the time and give you insight to how you were thinking/feeling. For best results, use a quote you really *feel* deep in your bones, and not just some Instagram tagline.

I know this may feel a tad repetitive but I can't overstate the importance of reflection when it comes to wellbeing. To best direct where you want to go, first you have to know where you have come from - there goes your first quote if you can't think of one.

Chapter Seven - References

1. Leydesdorff, L. (1998). Theories of citation? *Scientometrics, 43*(1), 5–25. https://doi.org/10.1007/BF02458391
2. Fuller, P. M., Gooley, J. J., & Saper, C. B. (2006). Neurobiology of the Sleep-Wake Cycle: Sleep Architecture, Circadian Regulation, and Regulatory Feedback. *Journal of Biological Rhythms, 21*(6), 482–493. https://doi.org/10.1177/0748730406294627
3. Deatherage, J. R., Roden, R. D., & Zouhary, K. (2009). Normal Sleep Architecture. *Seminars in Orthodontics, 15*(2), 86–87. https://doi.org/10.1053/j.sodo.2009.01.002
4. Walker, M. (2017). Why We Sleep: Unlocking the Power of Sleep and Dreams. United Kingdom: Scribner.
5. Coomans, C. P., Ramkisoensing, A., & Meijer, J. H. (2015). The suprachiasmatic nuclei as a seasonal clock. *Frontiers in Neuroendocrinology, 37*, 29–42. https://doi.org/10.1016/j.yfrne.2014.11.002
6. Gaus, S. E., Strecker, R. E., Tate, B. A., Parker, R. A., & Saper, C. B. (2002). Ventrolateral preoptic nucleus contains sleep-active, galaninergic neurons in multiple mammalian species. *Neuroscience, 115*(1), 285–294. https://doi.org/10.1016/S0306-4522(02)00308-1
7. Huang, Z.-L., Urade, Y., & Hayaishi, O. (2011). The Role of Adenosine in the Regulation of Sleep. *Current Topics in Medicinal Chemistry, 11*(8), 1047–1057. https://doi.org/10.2174/156802611795347654
8. Phillips, A. J. K., & Robinson, P. A. (2007). A Quantitative Model of Sleep-Wake Dynamics Based on the Physiology of the Brainstem Ascending Arousal System. *Journal of Biological Rhythms, 22*(2), 167–179. https://doi.org/10.1177/0748730406297512

9. Muzur, A., Pace-Schott, E. F., & Hobson, J. A. (2002). The prefrontal cortex in sleep. *Trends in Cognitive Sciences*, *6*(11), 475–481. https://doi.org/10.1016/S1364-6613(02)01992-7

10. Porter, V. R., Buxton, W. G., & Avidan, A. Y. (2015). Sleep, Cognition and Dementia. *Current Psychiatry Reports*, *17*(12), 97. https://doi.org/10.1007/s11920-015-0631-8

11. Sutanto, C. N., Loh, W. W., & Kim, J. E. (2022). The impact of tryptophan supplementation on sleep quality: a systematic review, meta-analysis, and meta-regression. *Nutrition Reviews*, *80*(2), 306–316. https://doi.org/10.1093/nutrit/nuab027

12. Choi, K., Lee, Y. J., Park, S., Je, N. K., & Suh, H. S. (2022). Efficacy of melatonin for chronic insomnia: Systematic reviews and meta-analyses. *Sleep Medicine Reviews*, *66*, 101692. https://doi.org/10.1016/j.smrv.2022.101692

13. Morales, J., Yáñez, A., Fernández-González, L., Montesinos-Magraner, L., Marco-Ahulló, A., Solana-Tramunt, M., & Calvete, E. (2019). Stress and autonomic response to sleep deprivation in medical residents: A comparative cross-sectional study. *PLOS ONE*, *14*(4), e0214858. https://doi.org/10.1371/journal.pone.0214858

14. Brum, M. C. B., Dantas Filho, F. F., Schnorr, C. C., Bertoletti, O. A., Bottega, G. B., & da Costa Rodrigues, T. (2020). Night shift work, short sleep and obesity. *Diabetology & Metabolic Syndrome*, *12*(1), 13. https://doi.org/10.1186/s13098-020-0524-9

15. Saidi, O., Rochette, E., del Sordo, G., Peyrel, P., Salles, J., Doré, E., Merlin, E., Walrand, S., & Duché, P. (2022). Isocaloric Diets with Different Protein-Carbohydrate Ratios: The Effect on Sleep, Melatonin Secretion and Subsequent Nutritional Response in Healthy Young Men. *Nutrients*, *14*(24), 5299. https://doi.org/10.3390/nu14245299

16. Fernández-Real, J.-M., & Ricart, W. (1999). Insulin resistance and inflammation in an evolutionary perspective: the contribution of cytokine genotype/phenotype to thriftiness. *Diabetologia*, *42*(11), 1367–1374. https://doi.org/10.1007/s001250051451

17. Benjamins, J. S., Hooge, I. T. C., Benedict, C., Smeets, P. A. M., & van der Laan, L. N. (2021). The influence of acute partial sleep deprivation on liking, choosing and consuming high- and low-

energy foods. *Food Quality and Preference, 88*, 104074. https://doi.org/10.1016/j.foodqual.2020.104074

18. Kuna, S. T., Reboussin, D. M., Strotmeyer, E. S., Millman, R. P., Zammit, G., Walkup, M. P., Wadden, T. A., Wing, R. R., Pi-Sunyer, F. X., Spira, A. P., Foster, G. D., Freeman, J., Patricio, J., Sifferman, A., McGuckin, B., Krauthamer-Ewing, S., Jones-Parker, M., Anastasi, M., Staley, B., … vander Veur, S. (2021). Effects of Weight Loss on Obstructive Sleep Apnea Severity. Ten-Year Results of the Sleep AHEAD Study. *American Journal of Respiratory and Critical Care Medicine, 203*(2), 221–229. https://doi.org/10.1164/rccm.201912-2511OC

19. Shibli, F., Skeans, J., Yamasaki, T., & Fass, R. (2020). Nocturnal Gastroesophageal Reflux Disease (GERD) and Sleep. *Journal of Clinical Gastroenterology, 54*(8), 663–674. https://doi.org/10.1097/MCG.0000000000001382

20. Mumtaz, H., Ghafoor, B., Saghir, H., Tariq, M., Dahar, K., Ali, S. H., Waheed, S. T., & Syed, A. A. (2022). Association of Vitamin B12 deficiency with long-term PPIs use: A cohort study. *Annals of Medicine and Surgery, 82*, 104762. https://doi.org/10.1016/j.amsu.2022.104762

21. Tu, Q., Heitkemper, M. M., Jarrett, M. E., & Buchanan, D. T. (2017). Sleep disturbances in irritable bowel syndrome: a systematic review. *Neurogastroenterology & Motility, 29*(3), e12946. https://doi.org/10.1111/nmo.12946

22. Lashley, Felissa R. RN, PhD, ACRN, FACMG, FAAN. A Review of Sleep in Selected Immune and Autoimmune Disorders. Holistic Nursing Practice 17(2):p 65-80, March 2003

23. Holt, G. R. (2019). Are SSRIs more effective than placebo in patients with major depressive disorder? *Evidence-Based Practice, 22*(4), 4–4. https://doi.org/10.1097/EBP.0000000000000372

24. O'Mahony, S. M., Clarke, G., Borre, Y. E., Dinan, T. G., & Cryan, J. F. (2015). Serotonin, tryptophan metabolism and the brain-gut-microbiome axis. Behavioural Brain Research, 277, 32–48. https://doi.org/10.1016/j.bbr.2014.07.027

25. Boland, E. M., Kelley, N. J., Chat, I. K.-Y., Zinbarg, R., Craske, M. G., Bookheimer, S., & Nusslock, R. (2022). Poor sleep quality is

significantly associated with effort but not temporal discounting of monetary rewards. Motivation Science, 8(1), 70–76. https://doi.org/10.1037/mot0000258

26. Curtis, B. J., Williams, P. G., & Anderson, J. S. (2018). Objective cognitive functioning in self-reported habitual short sleepers not reporting daytime dysfunction: examination of impulsivity via delay discounting. Sleep, 41(9). https://doi.org/10.1093/sleep/zsy115

27. Bernert, R. A., & Joiner, T. E. (2007). Sleep disturbances and suicide risk: A review of the literature. Neuropsychiatric Disease and Treatment, 3(6), 735–743. https://doi.org/10.2147/ndt.s1248

28. Alimoradi, Z., Lin, C.-Y., Broström, A., Bülow, P. H., Bajalan, Z., Griffiths, M. D., Ohayon, M. M., & Pakpour, A. H. (2019). Internet addiction and sleep problems: A systematic review and meta-analysis. Sleep Medicine Reviews, 47, 51–61. https://doi.org/10.1016/j.smrv.2019.06.004

29. Gillin, J. C. (1998). Are sleep disturbances risk factors for anxiety, depressive and addictive disorders? Acta Psychiatrica Scandinavica, 98(s393), 39–43. https://doi.org/10.1111/j.1600-0447.1998.tb05965.x

30. Mujica, A., Crowell, C., Villano, M., & Uddin, K. (2022). ADDICTION BY DESIGN: Some Dimensions and Challenges of Excessive Social Media Use. Medical Research Archives, 10(2). https://doi.org/10.18103/mra.v10i2.2677

31. Ribeiro, J. A., & Sebastião, A. M. (2010). Caffeine and Adenosine. Journal of Alzheimer's Disease, 20(s1), S3–S15. https://doi.org/10.3233/JAD-2010-1379

32. Angarita, G. A., Emadi, N., Hodges, S., & Morgan, P. T. (2016). Sleep abnormalities associated with alcohol, cannabis, cocaine, and opiate use: a comprehensive review. Addiction Science & Clinical Practice, 11(1), 9. https://doi.org/10.1186/s13722-016-0056-7

33. Naiman, R. (2017). Dreamless: the silent epidemic of REM sleep loss. Annals of the New York Academy of Sciences, 1406(1), 77–85. https://doi.org/10.1111/nyas.13447

34. Manber, R., Bootzin, R. R., Acebo, C., & Carskadon, M. A. (1996). The effects of regularizing sleep-wake schedules on daytime sleepiness. Sleep, 19(5), 432-441.
35. Mindell, J. A., & Williamson, A. A. (2018). Benefits of a bedtime routine in young children: Sleep, development, and beyond. Sleep medicine reviews, 40, 93-108.
36. Zhang, N., Cao, B., & Zhu, Y. (2019). Effects of pre-sleep thermal environment on human thermal state and sleep quality. Building and Environment, 148, 600-608.
37. Lastella, M., O'Mullan, C., Paterson, J. L., & Reynolds, A. C. (2019). Sex and sleep: perceptions of sex as a sleep promoting behavior in the general adult population. Frontiers in public health, 33.
38. Oesterling, C. F., Borg, C., Juhola, E., & Lancel, M. (2023). The influence of sexual activity on sleep: A diary study. Journal of Sleep Research, e13814.
39. Scullin, M. K., Krueger, M. L., Ballard, H. K., Pruett, N., & Bliwise, D. L. (2018). The effects of bedtime writing on difficulty falling asleep: A polysomnographic study comparing to-do lists and completed activity lists. Journal of Experimental Psychology: General, 147(1), 139.
40. Elbourne, S. (2022). Promoting comfort and sleep. In Developing Practical Nursing Skills (pp. 389-418). Routledge.
41. Emmons, R. A., & McCullough, M. E. (2003). Counting blessings versus burdens: an experimental investigation of gratitude and subjective well-being in daily life. Journal of personality and social psychology, 84(2), 377.
42. Dentico, D., Ferrarelli, F., Riedner, B. A., Smith, R., Zennig, C., Lutz, A., ... & Davidson, R. J. (2016). Short meditation trainings enhance non-REM sleep low-frequency oscillations. PLoS One, 11(2), e0148961.

SLEEP SHEETS

BEDTIME: WAKING TIME: APPROX. SLEEP HOURS:

BEDTIME ROUTINE

ACHIEVED
TODAY

1.
2.
3.

MUST DO
TOMORROW

1.
2.
3.

TODAY
I'M GRATEFUL FOR

BRAIN DUMP
AND "DONT FORGETS"

SLEEP HYGINE CHECKS
IF APPLICABLE

1.
2.
3.

DOODLE SPACE

LOVING-KINDNESS

TODAYS QUOTABLE

Sleep Sheets

BEDTIME: WAKING TIME: APPROX. SLEEP HOURS:

BEDTIME ROUTINE

ACHIEVED
TODAY
1
2
3

MUST DO
TOMORROW
1 ○
2 ○
3 ○

TODAY
I'M GRATEFUL FOR

BRAIN DUMP
AND "DONT FORGETS"

SLEEP HYGIENE CHECKS
IF APPLICABLE
1 ○
2 ○
3 ○

DOODLE SPACE

LOVING-KINDNESS

TODAYS QUOTABLE

Sleep Sheets

BEDTIME: WAKING TIME: APPROX. SLEEP HOURS:

BEDTIME ROUTINE

ACHIEVED
TODAY
1.
2.
3.

MUST DO
TOMORROW
1.
2.
3.

TODAY
I'M GRATEFUL FOR

BRAIN DUMP
AND "DONT FORGETS"

SLEEP HYGIENE CHECKS
IF APPLICABLE
1.
2.
3.

DOODLE SPACE

LOVING-KINDNESS

TODAYS QUOTABLE

Sleep Sheets

BEDTIME: _____ WAKING TIME: _____ APPROX. SLEEP HOURS: _____

BEDTIME ROUTINE

ACHIEVED
TODAY
1. _____
2. _____
3. _____

MUST DO
TOMORROW
1. _____ ○
2. _____ ○
3. _____ ○

TODAY
I'M GRATEFUL FOR

BRAIN DUMP
AND "DONT FORGETS"

SLEEP HYGINE CHECKS
IF APPLICABLE
1. _____ ○
2. _____ ○
3. _____ ○

DOODLE SPACE

LOVING-KINDNESS

TODAYS QUOTABLE

SLEEP SHEETS

BEDTIME: WAKING TIME: APPROX. SLEEP HOURS:

BEDTIME ROUTINE

ACHIEVED
TODAY

1
2
3

MUST DO
TOMORROW

1
2
3

TODAY
I'M GRATEFUL FOR

BRAIN DUMP
AND "DONT FORGETS"

SLEEP HYGINE CHECKS
IF APPLICABLE

1
2
3

DOODLE SPACE

LOVING-KINDNESS

TODAYS QUOTABLE

Sleep Sheets

BEDTIME: _____ WAKING TIME: _____ APPROX. SLEEP HOURS: _____

BEDTIME ROUTINE

ACHIEVED
TODAY

1 ....
2 ....
3 ....

MUST DO
TOMORROW

1 .... ○
2 .... ○
3 .... ○

TODAY
I'M GRATEFUL FOR

BRAIN DUMP
AND "DONT FORGETS"

SLEEP HYGIENE CHECKS
IF APPLICABLE

1 .... ○
2 .... ○
3 .... ○

DOODLE SPACE

LOVING-KINDNESS

TODAYS QUOTABLE

Sleep Sheets

BEDTIME: WAKING TIME: APPROX. SLEEP HOURS:

BEDTIME ROUTINE

ACHIEVED
TODAY
1.
2.
3.

MUST DO
TOMORROW
1.
2.
3.

TODAY
I'M GRATEFUL FOR

BRAIN DUMP
AND "DONT FORGETS"

SLEEP HYGINE CHECKS
IF APPLICABLE
1.
2.
3.

DOODLE SPACE

LOVING-KINDNESS

TODAYS QUOTABLE

Sleep Sheets

BEDTIME: WAKING TIME: APPROX. SLEEP HOURS:

BEDTIME ROUTINE

ACHIEVED TODAY
1
2
3

MUST DO TOMORROW
1 ○
2 ○
3 ○

TODAY I'M GRATEFUL FOR

BRAIN DUMP
AND "DONT FORGETS"

SLEEP HYGINE CHECKS
IF APPLICABLE
1 ○
2 ○
3 ○

DOODLE SPACE

LOVING-KINDNESS

TODAYS QUOTABLE

Sleep Sheets

BEDTIME: WAKING TIME: APPROX. SLEEP HOURS:

BEDTIME ROUTINE

ACHIEVED TODAY
1.
2.
3.

MUST DO TOMORROW
1.
2.
3.

TODAY I'M GRATEFUL FOR

BRAIN DUMP
AND "DONT FORGETS"

SLEEP HYGINE CHECKS
IF APPLICABLE
1.
2.
3.

DOODLE SPACE

LOVING-KINDNESS

TODAYS QUOTABLE

Sleep Sheets

BEDTIME: WAKING TIME: APPROX. SLEEP HOURS:

BEDTIME ROUTINE

ACHIEVED
TODAY
1.
2.
3.

MUST DO
TOMORROW
1. ○
2. ○
3. ○

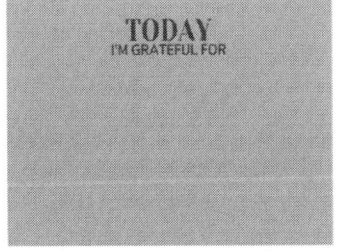

TODAY
I'M GRATEFUL FOR

BRAIN DUMP
AND "DONT FORGETS"

SLEEP HYGINE CHECKS
IF APPLICABLE
1. ○
2. ○
3. ○

DOODLE SPACE

LOVING-KINDNESS

TODAYS QUOTABLE

Sleep Sheets

BEDTIME: WAKING TIME: APPROX. SLEEP HOURS:

BEDTIME ROUTINE

ACHIEVED
TODAY
1.
2.
3.

MUST DO
TOMORROW
1. ○
2. ○
3. ○

TODAY
I'M GRATEFUL FOR

BRAIN DUMP
AND "DONT FORGETS"

SLEEP HYGINE CHECKS
IF APPLICABLE
1. ○
2. ○
3. ○

DOODLE SPACE

LOVING-KINDNESS

TODAYS QUOTABLE

SLEEP SHEETS

BEDTIME: WAKING TIME: APPROX. SLEEP HOURS:

BEDTIME ROUTINE

ACHIEVED
TODAY

1
2
3

MUST DO
TOMORROW

1
2
3

TODAY
I'M GRATEFUL FOR

BRAIN DUMP
AND "DONT FORGETS"

SLEEP HYGINE CHECKS
IF APPLICABLE

1
2
3

DOODLE SPACE

LOVING-KINDNESS

TODAYS QUOTABLE

SLEEP SHEETS

BEDTIME: WAKING TIME: APPROX. SLEEP HOURS:

BEDTIME ROUTINE

ACHIEVED
TODAY
1
2
3

MUST DO
TOMORROW
1
2
3

TODAY
I'M GRATEFUL FOR

BRAIN DUMP
AND "DONT FORGETS"

SLEEP HYGINE CHECKS
IF APPLICABLE
1
2
3

DOODLE SPACE

LOVING-KINDNESS

TODAYS QUOTABLE

Sleep Sheets

BEDTIME: _____ WAKING TIME: _____ APPROX. SLEEP HOURS: _____

BEDTIME ROUTINE

ACHIEVED TODAY
1. _____
2. _____
3. _____

MUST DO TOMORROW
1. _____ ○
2. _____ ○
3. _____ ○

TODAY I'M GRATEFUL FOR

BRAIN DUMP
AND "DONT FORGETS"

SLEEP HYGINE CHECKS
IF APPLICABLE
1. _____ ○
2. _____ ○
3. _____ ○

DOODLE SPACE

LOVING-KINDNESS

TODAYS QUOTABLE

Sleep Sheets

BEDTIME: **WAKING TIME:** **APPROX. SLEEP HOURS:**

BEDTIME ROUTINE

ACHIEVED
TODAY

1
2
3

MUST DO
TOMORROW

1
2
3

TODAY
I'M GRATEFUL FOR

BRAIN DUMP
AND "DONT FORGETS"

SLEEP HYGINE CHECKS
IF APPLICABLE

1
2
3

DOODLE SPACE

LOVING-KINDNESS

TODAYS QUOTABLE

Sleep Sheets

BEDTIME:　　　WAKING TIME:　　　APPROX. SLEEP HOURS:

BEDTIME ROUTINE

ACHIEVED
TODAY

1
2
3

MUST DO
TOMORROW

1
2
3

TODAY
I'M GRATEFUL FOR

BRAIN DUMP
AND "DONT FORGETS"

SLEEP HYGINE CHECKS
IF APPLICABLE

1
2
3

DOODLE SPACE

LOVING-KINDNESS

TODAYS QUOTABLE

SLEEP SHEETS

BEDTIME: WAKING TIME: APPROX. SLEEP HOURS:

BEDTIME ROUTINE

ACHIEVED
TODAY

1
2
3

MUST DO
TOMORROW

1
2
3

TODAY
I'M GRATEFUL FOR

BRAIN DUMP
AND "DONT FORGETS"

SLEEP HYGINE CHECKS
IF APPLICABLE

1
2
3

DOODLE SPACE

LOVING-KINDNESS

TODAYS QUOTABLE

Sleep Sheets

BEDTIME: WAKING TIME: APPROX. SLEEP HOURS:

BEDTIME ROUTINE

ACHIEVED
TODAY

1
2
3

MUST DO
TOMORROW

1
2
3

TODAY
I'M GRATEFUL FOR

BRAIN DUMP
AND "DONT FORGETS"

SLEEP HYGINE CHECKS
IF APPLICABLE

1
2
3

DOODLE SPACE

LOVING-KINDNESS

TODAYS QUOTABLE

Sleep Sheets

BEDTIME: **WAKING TIME:**   **APPROX. SLEEP HOURS:**

BEDTIME ROUTINE

ACHIEVED
TODAY

1.
2.
3.

MUST DO
TOMORROW

1.
2.
3.

TODAY
I'M GRATEFUL FOR

BRAIN DUMP
AND "DONT FORGETS"

SLEEP HYGINE CHECKS
IF APPLICABLE

1.
2.
3.

DOODLE SPACE

LOVING-KINDNESS

TODAYS QUOTABLE

Sleep Sheets

BEDTIME: WAKING TIME: APPROX. SLEEP HOURS:

BEDTIME ROUTINE

ACHIEVED
TODAY

1
2
3

MUST DO
TOMORROW

1
2
3

TODAY
I'M GRATEFUL FOR

BRAIN DUMP
AND "DONT FORGETS"

SLEEP HYGINE CHECKS
IF APPLICABLE

1
2
3

DOODLE SPACE

LOVING KINDNESS

TODAYS QUOTABLE

SLEEP SHEETS

BEDTIME: _____   WAKING TIME: _____   APPROX. SLEEP HOURS: _____

BEDTIME ROUTINE

ACHIEVED
TODAY
1. _____
2. _____
3. _____

MUST DO
TOMORROW
1. _____ ○
2. _____ ○
3. _____ ○

TODAY
I'M GRATEFUL FOR

BRAIN DUMP
AND "DONT FORGETS"

SLEEP HYGINE CHECKS
IF APPLICABLE
1. _____ ○
2. _____ ○
3. _____ ○

DOODLE SPACE

LOVING-KINDNESS

TODAYS QUOTABLE

SLEEP SHEETS

BEDTIME:　　　　　WAKING TIME:　　　　　APPROX. SLEEP HOURS:

BEDTIME ROUTINE

ACHIEVED
TODAY

1
2
3

MUST DO
TOMORROW

1
2
3

TODAY
I'M GRATEFUL FOR

BRAIN DUMP
AND "DONT FORGETS"

SLEEP HYGINE CHECKS
IF APPLICABLE

1
2
3

DOODLE SPACE

LOVING-KINDNESS

TODAYS QUOTABLE

Sleep Sheets

BEDTIME: _____ WAKING TIME: _____ APPROX. SLEEP HOURS: _____

BEDTIME ROUTINE

ACHIEVED
TODAY
1. _____
2. _____
3. _____

MUST DO
TOMORROW
1. _____ ○
2. _____ ○
3. _____ ○

TODAY
I'M GRATEFUL FOR

BRAIN DUMP
AND "DONT FORGETS"

SLEEP HYGINE CHECKS
IF APPLICABLE
1. _____ ○
2. _____ ○
3. _____ ○

DOODLE SPACE

LOVING-KINDNESS

TODAYS QUOTABLE

Sleep Sheets

BEDTIME: WAKING TIME: APPROX. SLEEP HOURS:

BEDTIME ROUTINE

ACHIEVED
TODAY

1.
2.
3.

MUST DO
TOMORROW

1.
2.
3.

TODAY
I'M GRATEFUL FOR

BRAIN DUMP
AND "DONT FORGETS"

SLEEP HYGINE CHECKS
IF APPLICABLE

1.
2.
3.

DOODLE SPACE

LOVING-KINDNESS

TODAYS QUOTABLE

SLEEP SHEETS

BEDTIME: WAKING TIME: APPROX. SLEEP HOURS:

BEDTIME ROUTINE

ACHIEVED
TODAY
1.
2.
3.

MUST DO
TOMORROW
1.
2.
3.

TODAY
I'M GRATEFUL FOR

BRAIN DUMP
AND "DONT FORGETS"

SLEEP HYGINE CHECKS
IF APPLICABLE
1.
2.
3.

DOODLE SPACE

LOVING-KINDNESS

TODAYS QUOTABLE

Sleep Sheets

BEDTIME: WAKING TIME: APPROX. SLEEP HOURS:

BEDTIME ROUTINE

ACHIEVED
TODAY
1
2
3

MUST DO
TOMORROW
1
2
3

TODAY
I'M GRATEFUL FOR

BRAIN DUMP
AND "DONT FORGETS"

SLEEP HYGINE CHECKS
IF APPLICABLE
1
2
3

DOODLE SPACE

LOVING-KINDNESS

TODAYS QUOTABLE

Sleep Sheets

BEDTIME: WAKING TIME: APPROX. SLEEP HOURS:

Bedtime Routine

Achieved
Today
1.
2.
3.

Must Do
Tomorrow
1.
2.
3.

Today
I'm Grateful For

Brain Dump
And "Don't Forgets"

Sleep Hygiene Checks
If Applicable
1.
2.
3.

Doodle Space

Loving-Kindness

Todays Quotable

SLEEP SHEETS

BEDTIME: WAKING TIME: APPROX. SLEEP HOURS:

BEDTIME ROUTINE

ACHIEVED
TODAY
1.
2.
3.

MUST DO
TOMORROW
1.
2.
3.

TODAY
I'M GRATEFUL FOR

BRAIN DUMP
AND "DONT FORGETS"

SLEEP HYGINE CHECKS
IF APPLICABLE
1.
2.
3.

DOODLE SPACE

LOVING-KINDNESS

TODAYS QUOTABLE

Sleep Sheets

BEDTIME: _____ WAKING TIME: _____ APPROX. SLEEP HOURS: _____

BEDTIME ROUTINE

ACHIEVED
TODAY

1 _____
2 _____
3 _____

MUST DO
TOMORROW

1 _____ ○
2 _____ ○
3 _____ ○

TODAY
I'M GRATEFUL FOR

BRAIN DUMP
AND "DONT FORGETS"

SLEEP HYGINE CHECKS
IF APPLICABLE

1 _____ ○
2 _____ ○
3 _____ ○

DOODLE SPACE

LOVING-KINDNESS

TODAYS QUOTABLE

Sleep Sheets

BEDTIME:　　　　WAKING TIME:　　　　APPROX. SLEEP HOURS:

BEDTIME ROUTINE

ACHIEVED
TODAY
1
2
3

MUST DO
TOMORROW
1
2
3

TODAY
I'M GRATEFUL FOR

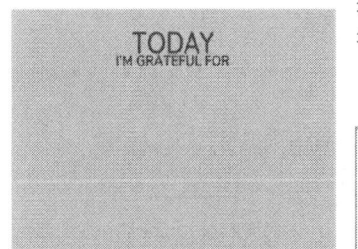

BRAIN DUMP
AND "DONT FORGETS"

SLEEP HYGINE CHECKS
IF APPLICABLE
1
2
3

DOODLE SPACE

LOVING-KINDNESS

TODAYS QUOTABLE

SLEEP SHEETS

BEDTIME: WAKING TIME: APPROX. SLEEP HOURS:

BEDTIME ROUTINE

ACHIEVED
TODAY
1
2
3

MUST DO
TOMORROW
1
2
3

TODAY
I'M GRATEFUL FOR

BRAIN DUMP
AND "DONT FORGETS"

SLEEP HYGINE CHECKS
IF APPLICABLE
1
2
3

DOODLE SPACE

LOVING-KINDNESS

TODAYS QUOTABLE

Sleep Sheets

BEDTIME: _____ WAKING TIME: _____ APPROX. SLEEP HOURS: _____

BEDTIME ROUTINE

ACHIEVED
TODAY

1. _____
2. _____
3. _____

MUST DO
TOMORROW

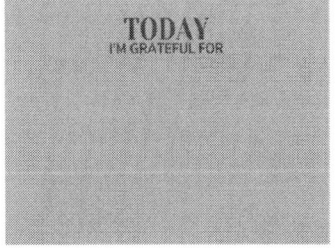

1. _____ ○
2. _____ ○
3. _____ ○

TODAY
I'M GRATEFUL FOR

BRAIN DUMP
AND "DONT FORGETS"

SLEEP HYGINE CHECKS
IF APPLICABLE

1. _____ ○
2. _____ ○
3. _____ ○

DOODLE SPACE

LOVING-KINDNESS

TODAYS QUOTABLE

Sleep Sheets

BEDTIME: WAKING TIME: APPROX. SLEEP HOURS:

BEDTIME ROUTINE

ACHIEVED
TODAY
1.
2.
3.

MUST DO
TOMORROW
1. ○
2. ○
3. ○

TODAY
I'M GRATEFUL FOR

BRAIN DUMP
AND "DONT FORGETS"

SLEEP HYGIENE CHECKS
IF APPLICABLE
1. ○
2. ○
3. ○

DOODLE SPACE

LOVING-KINDNESS

TODAYS QUOTABLE

Sleep Sheets

BEDTIME: WAKING TIME: APPROX. SLEEP HOURS:

BEDTIME ROUTINE

ACHIEVED
TODAY

1
2
3

MUST DO
TOMORROW

1
2
3

TODAY
I'M GRATEFUL FOR

BRAIN DUMP
AND "DONT FORGETS"

SLEEP HYGINE CHECKS
IF APPLICABLE

1
2
3

DOODLE SPACE

LOVING-KINDNESS

TODAYS QUOTABLE

Sleep Sheets

BEDTIME: WAKING TIME: APPROX. SLEEP HOURS:

BEDTIME ROUTINE

ACHIEVED
TODAY
1
2
3

MUST DO
TOMORROW
1
2
3

TODAY
I'M GRATEFUL FOR

BRAIN DUMP
AND "DONT FORGETS"

SLEEP HYGINE CHECKS
IF APPLICABLE
1
2
3

DOODLE SPACE

LOVING-KINDNESS

TODAYS QUOTABLE

Sleep Sheets

BEDTIME: WAKING TIME: APPROX. SLEEP HOURS:

BEDTIME ROUTINE

ACHIEVED
TODAY

1
2
3

MUST DO
TOMORROW

1
2
3

TODAY
I'M GRATEFUL FOR

BRAIN DUMP
AND "DONT FORGETS"

SLEEP HYGINE CHECKS
IF APPLICABLE

1
2
3

DOODLE SPACE

LOVING-KINDNESS

TODAYS QUOTABLE

SLEEP SHEETS

BEDTIME: WAKING TIME: APPROX SLEEP HOURS:

BEDTIME ROUTINE

ACHIEVED
TODAY

1
2
3

MUST DO
TOMORROW

1 ○
2 ○
3 ○

TODAY
I'M GRATEFUL FOR

BRAIN DUMP
AND "DONT FORGETS"

SLEEP HYGINE CHECKS
IF APPLICABLE

1 ○
2 ○
3 ○

DOODLE SPACE

LOVING-KINDNESS

TODAYS QUOTABLE

Sleep Sheets

BEDTIME: WAKING TIME: APPROX. SLEEP HOURS:

BEDTIME ROUTINE

ACHIEVED
TODAY

1
2
3

MUST DO
TOMORROW

1
2
3

TODAY
I'M GRATEFUL FOR

BRAIN DUMP
AND "DONT FORGETS"

SLEEP HYGINE CHECKS
IF APPLICABLE

1
2
3

DOODLE SPACE

LOVING-KINDNESS

TODAYS QUOTABLE

Sleep Sheets

BEDTIME: WAKING TIME: APPROX. SLEEP HOURS:

BEDTIME ROUTINE

ACHIEVED
TODAY
1
2
3

MUST DO
TOMORROW
1
2
3

TODAY
I'M GRATEFUL FOR

BRAIN DUMP
AND "DONT FORGETS"

SLEEP HYGINE CHECKS
IF APPLICABLE
1
2
3

DOODLE SPACE

LOVING-KINDNESS

TODAYS QUOTABLE

SLEEP SHEETS

BEDTIME: WAKING TIME: APPROX. SLEEP HOURS:

BEDTIME ROUTINE

ACHIEVED
TODAY
1
2
3

MUST DO
TOMORROW
1
2
3

TODAY
I'M GRATEFUL FOR

BRAIN DUMP
AND "DONT FORGETS"

SLEEP HYGINE CHECKS
IF APPLICABLE
1
2
3

DOODLE SPACE

LOVING-KINDNESS

TODAYS QUOTABLE

Sleep Sheets

BEDTIME: WAKING TIME: APPROX. SLEEP HOURS:

BEDTIME ROUTINE

ACHIEVED
TODAY
1
2
3

MUST DO
TOMORROW
1
2
3

TODAY
I'M GRATEFUL FOR

BRAIN DUMP
AND "DONT FORGETS"

SLEEP HYGINE CHECKS
IF APPLICABLE
1
2
3

DOODLE SPACE

LOVING-KINDNESS

TODAYS QUOTABLE

Sleep Sheets

BEDTIME: WAKING TIME: APPROX. SLEEP HOURS:

BEDTIME ROUTINE

ACHIEVED
TODAY
1
2
3

MUST DO
TOMORROW
1
2
3

TODAY
I'M GRATEFUL FOR

BRAIN DUMP
AND "DONT FORGETS"

SLEEP HYGINE CHECKS
IF APPLICABLE
1
2
3

DOODLE SPACE

LOVING-KINDNESS

TODAYS QUOTABLE

Sleep Sheets

BEDTIME: WAKING TIME: APPROX. SLEEP HOURS:

BEDTIME ROUTINE

ACHIEVED
TODAY
1.
2.
3.

MUST DO
TOMORROW
1. ○
2. ○
3. ○

TODAY
I'M GRATEFUL FOR

BRAIN DUMP
AND "DONT FORGETS"

SLEEP HYGINE CHECKS
IF APPLICABLE
1. ○
2. ○
3. ○

DOODLE SPACE

LOVING-KINDNESS

TODAYS QUOTABLE

SLEEP SHEETS

BEDTIME: WAKING TIME: APPROX. SLEEP HOURS:

BEDTIME ROUTINE

ACHIEVED
TODAY

1
2
3

MUST DO
TOMORROW

1
2
3

TODAY
I'M GRATEFUL FOR

BRAIN DUMP
AND "DONT FORGETS"

SLEEP HYGINE CHECKS
IF APPLICABLE

1
2
3

DOODLE SPACE

LOVING-KINDNESS

TODAYS QUOTABLE

Sleep Sheets

BEDTIME: WAKING TIME: APPROX. SLEEP HOURS:

BEDTIME ROUTINE

ACHIEVED TODAY
1.
2.
3.

MUST DO TOMORROW
1. ○
2. ○
3. ○

TODAY I'M GRATEFUL FOR

BRAIN DUMP
AND "DONT FORGETS"

SLEEP HYGIENE CHECKS
IF APPLICABLE
1. ○
2. ○
3. ○

DOODLE SPACE

LOVING KINDNESS

TODAYS QUOTABLE

Sleep Sheets

BEDTIME: WAKING TIME: APPROX. SLEEP HOURS:

BEDTIME ROUTINE

ACHIEVED
TODAY

1
2
3

MUST DO
TOMORROW

1
2
3

TODAY
I'M GRATEFUL FOR

BRAIN DUMP
AND "DONT FORGETS"

SLEEP HYGINE CHECKS
IF APPLICABLE

1
2
3

DOODLE SPACE

LOVING-KINDNESS

TODAYS QUOTABLE

SLEEP SHEETS

BEDTIME: WAKING TIME: APPROX. SLEEP HOURS:

BEDTIME ROUTINE

ACHIEVED
TODAY
1
2
3

MUST DO
TOMORROW
1
2
3

TODAY
I'M GRATEFUL FOR

BRAIN DUMP
AND "DONT FORGETS"

SLEEP HYGINE CHECKS
IF APPLICABLE
1
2
3

DOODLE SPACE

LOVING-KINDNESS

TODAYS QUOTABLE

Sleep Sheets

BEDTIME: WAKING TIME: APPROX. SLEEP HOURS:

BEDTIME ROUTINE

ACHIEVED
TODAY

1
2
3

MUST DO
TOMORROW

1
2
3

TODAY
I'M GRATEFUL FOR

BRAIN DUMP
AND "DONT FORGETS"

SLEEP HYGINE CHECKS
IF APPLICABLE

1
2
3

DOODLE SPACE

LOVING-KINDNESS

TODAYS QUOTABLE

Sleep Sheets

BEDTIME: WAKING TIME: APPROX. SLEEP HOURS:

BEDTIME ROUTINE

ACHIEVED
TODAY

1.
2.
3.

MUST DO
TOMORROW

1. ○
2. ○
3. ○

TODAY
I'M GRATEFUL FOR

BRAIN DUMP
AND "DONT FORGETS"

SLEEP HYGINE CHECKS
IF APPLICABLE

1. ○
2. ○
3. ○

DOODLE SPACE

LOVING-KINDNESS

TODAYS QUOTABLE

Sleep Sheets

BEDTIME: WAKING TIME: APPROX. SLEEP HOURS:

BEDTIME ROUTINE

ACHIEVED
TODAY

1
2
3

MUST DO
TOMORROW

1
2
3

TODAY
I'M GRATEFUL FOR

BRAIN DUMP
AND "DONT FORGETS"

SLEEP HYGINE CHECKS
IF APPLICABLE

1
2
3

DOODLE SPACE

LOVING-KINDNESS

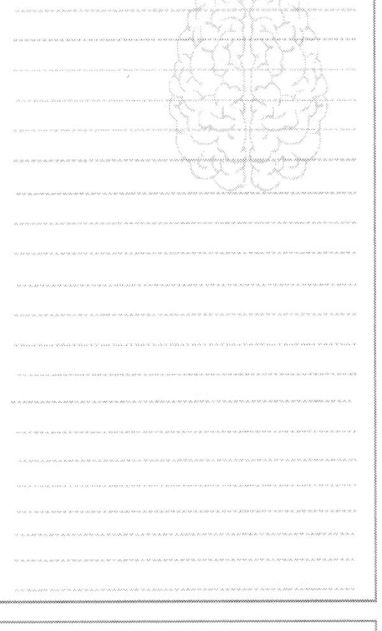

TODAYS QUOTABLE

Sleep Sheets

BEDTIME: WAKING TIME: APPROX. SLEEP HOURS:

BEDTIME ROUTINE

ACHIEVED TODAY

1.
2.
3.

MUST DO TOMORROW

1.
2.
3.

TODAY I'M GRATEFUL FOR

BRAIN DUMP
AND "DONT FORGETS"

SLEEP HYGINE CHECKS
IF APPLICABLE

1.
2.
3.

DOODLE SPACE

LOVING-KINDNESS

TODAYS QUOTABLE

SLEEP SHEETS

BEDTIME: WAKING TIME: APPROX. SLEEP HOURS:

BEDTIME ROUTINE

ACHIEVED
TODAY
1
2
3

MUST DO
TOMORROW
1
2
3

TODAY
I'M GRATEFUL FOR

BRAIN DUMP
AND "DONT FORGETS"

SLEEP HYGIENE CHECKS
IF APPLICABLE
1
2
3

DOODLE SPACE

LOVING-KINDNESS

TODAYS QUOTABLE

Sleep Sheets

BEDTIME: WAKING TIME: APPROX. SLEEP HOURS:

BEDTIME ROUTINE

ACHIEVED
TODAY
1.
2.
3.

MUST DO
TOMORROW
1.
2.
3.

TODAY
I'M GRATEFUL FOR

BRAIN DUMP
AND "DONT FORGETS"

SLEEP HYGINE CHECKS
IF APPLICABLE
1.
2.
3.

DOODLE SPACE

LOVING-KINDNESS

TODAYS QUOTABLE

SLEEP SHEETS

BEDTIME: WAKING TIME: APPROX. SLEEP HOURS:

BEDTIME ROUTINE

ACHIEVED
TODAY

1
2
3

MUST DO
TOMORROW

1
2
3

TODAY
I'M GRATEFUL FOR

BRAIN DUMP
AND "DONT FORGETS"

SLEEP HYGINE CHECKS
IF APPLICABLE

1
2
3

DOODLE SPACE

LOVING-KINDNESS

TODAYS QUOTABLE

Sleep Sheets

BEDTIME: WAKING TIME: APPROX. SLEEP HOURS:

BEDTIME ROUTINE

ACHIEVED
TODAY
1.
2.
3.

MUST DO
TOMORROW
1.
2.
3.

TODAY
I'M GRATEFUL FOR

BRAIN DUMP
AND "DONT FORGETS"

SLEEP HYGINE CHECKS
IF APPLICABLE
1.
2.
3.

DOODLE SPACE

LOVING-KINDNESS

TODAYS QUOTABLE

Sleep Sheets

BEDTIME: WAKING TIME: APPROX. SLEEP HOURS:

BEDTIME ROUTINE

ACHIEVED
TODAY

1
2
3

MUST DO
TOMORROW

1 ○
2 ○
3 ○

TODAY
I'M GRATEFUL FOR

BRAIN DUMP
AND "DONT FORGETS"

SLEEP HYGINE CHECKS
IF APPLICABLE

1 ○
2 ○
3 ○

DOODLE SPACE

LOVING-KINDNESS

TODAYS QUOTABLE

SLEEP SHEETS

BEDTIME: WAKING TIME: APPROX. SLEEP HOURS:

BEDTIME ROUTINE

ACHIEVED
TODAY
1
2
3

MUST DO
TOMORROW
1
2
3

TODAY
I'M GRATEFUL FOR

BRAIN DUMP
AND "DONT FORGETS"

SLEEP HYGINE CHECKS
IF APPLICABLE
1
2
3

DOODLE SPACE

LOVING-KINDNESS

TODAYS QUOTABLE

Sleep Sheets

BEDTIME: WAKING TIME: APPROX. SLEEP HOURS:

BEDTIME ROUTINE

ACHIEVED
TODAY

1
2
3

MUST DO
TOMORROW

1
2
3

TODAY
I'M GRATEFUL FOR

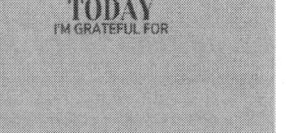

BRAIN DUMP
AND "DONT FORGETS"

SLEEP HYGINE CHECKS
IF APPLICABLE

1
2
3

DOODLE SPACE

LOVING-KINDNESS

TODAYS QUOTABLE

Sleep Sheets

BEDTIME: WAKING TIME: APPROX. SLEEP HOURS:

BEDTIME ROUTINE

ACHIEVED
TODAY

1.
2.
3.

MUST DO
TOMORROW

1.
2.
3.

TODAY
I'M GRATEFUL FOR

BRAIN DUMP
AND "DONT FORGETS"

SLEEP HYGINE CHECKS
IF APPLICABLE

1.
2.
3.

DOODLE SPACE

LOVING-KINDNESS

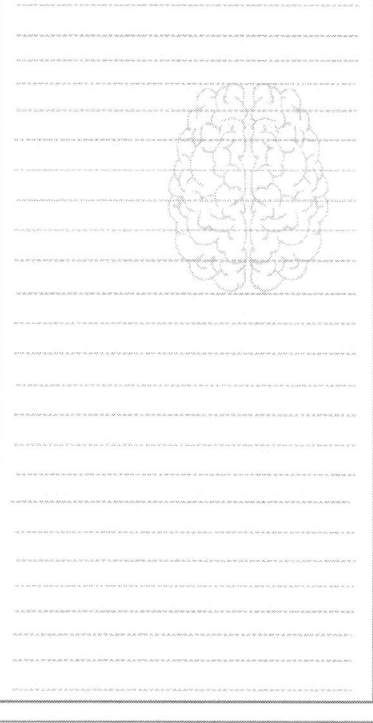

TODAYS QUOTABLE

Sleep Sheets

BEDTIME: WAKING TIME: APPROX. SLEEP HOURS:

BEDTIME ROUTINE

ACHIEVED
TODAY
1
2
3

MUST DO
TOMORROW
1
2
3

TODAY
I'M GRATEFUL FOR

BRAIN DUMP
AND "DONT FORGETS"

SLEEP HYGINE CHECKS
IF APPLICABLE
1
2
3

DOODLE SPACE

LOVING-KINDNESS

TODAYS QUOTABLE

Sleep Sheets

BEDTIME:　　　　WAKING TIME:　　　　APPROX SLEEP HOURS:

BEDTIME ROUTINE

ACHIEVED
TODAY
1
2
3

MUST DO
TOMORROW
1
2
3

TODAY
I'M GRATEFUL FOR

BRAIN DUMP
AND "DONT FORGETS"

SLEEP HYGINE CHECKS
IF APPLICABLE
1
2
3

DOODLE SPACE

LOVING-KINDNESS

TODAYS QUOTABLE

SLEEP SHEETS

BEDTIME:　　　　WAKING TIME:　　　　APPROX. SLEEP HOURS:

BEDTIME ROUTINE

ACHIEVED
TODAY

1
2
3

MUST DO
TOMORROW

1
2
3

TODAY
I'M GRATEFUL FOR

BRAIN DUMP
AND "DONT FORGETS"

SLEEP HYGINE CHECKS
IF APPLICABLE

1
2
3

DOODLE SPACE

LOVING-KINDNESS

TODAYS QUOTABLE

Sleep Sheets

BEDTIME: WAKING TIME: APPROX. SLEEP HOURS:

BEDTIME ROUTINE

ACHIEVED
TODAY
1
2
3

MUST DO
TOMORROW
1
2
3

TODAY
I'M GRATEFUL FOR

BRAIN DUMP
AND "DONT FORGETS"

SLEEP HYGINE CHECKS
IF APPLICABLE
1
2
3

DOODLE SPACE

LOVING-KINDNESS

TODAYS QUOTABLE

Sleep Sheets

BEDTIME: WAKING TIME: APPROX. SLEEP HOURS:

BEDTIME ROUTINE

ACHIEVED
TODAY

1.
2.
3.

MUST DO
TOMORROW

1. ○
2. ○
3. ○

TODAY
I'M GRATEFUL FOR

BRAIN DUMP
AND "DONT FORGETS"

SLEEP HYGIENE CHECKS
IF APPLICABLE

1. ○
2. ○
3. ○

DOODLE SPACE

LOVING-KINDNESS

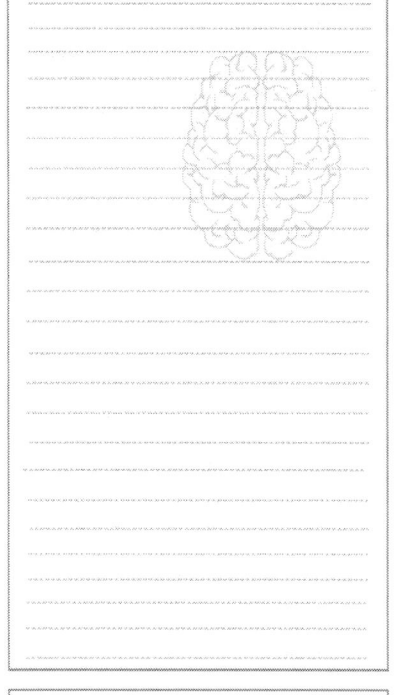

TODAYS QUOTABLE

SLEEP SHEETS

BEDTIME: WAKING TIME: APPROX. SLEEP HOURS:

BEDTIME ROUTINE

ACHIEVED
TODAY
1.
2.
3.

MUST DO
TOMORROW
1.
2.
3.

TODAY
I'M GRATEFUL FOR

BRAIN DUMP
AND "DONT FORGETS"

SLEEP HYGINE CHECKS
IF APPLICABLE
1.
2.
3.

DOODLE SPACE

LOVING-KINDNESS

TODAYS QUOTABLE

Sleep Sheets

BEDTIME: WAKING TIME: APPROX. SLEEP HOURS:

BEDTIME ROUTINE

ACHIEVED
TODAY
1.
2.
3.

MUST DO
TOMORROW
1. ○
2. ○
3. ○

TODAY
I'M GRATEFUL FOR

BRAIN DUMP
AND "DONT FORGETS"

SLEEP HYGINE CHECKS
IF APPLICABLE
1. ○
2. ○
3. ○

DOODLE SPACE

LOVING-KINDNESS

TODAYS QUOTABLE

Sleep Sheets

BEDTIME: WAKING TIME: APPROX. SLEEP HOURS:

BEDTIME ROUTINE

ACHIEVED
TODAY
1
2
3

MUST DO
TOMORROW
1
2
3

TODAY
I'M GRATEFUL FOR

BRAIN DUMP
AND "DONT FORGETS"

SLEEP HYGINE CHECKS
IF APPLICABLE
1
2
3

DOODLE SPACE

LOVING-KINDNESS

TODAYS QUOTABLE

Sleep Sheets

BEDTIME: WAKING TIME: APPROX. SLEEP HOURS:

BEDTIME ROUTINE

ACHIEVED
TODAY

1
2
3

MUST DO
TOMORROW

1
2
3

TODAY
I'M GRATEFUL FOR

BRAIN DUMP
AND "DONT FORGETS"

SLEEP HYGINE CHECKS
IF APPLICABLE

1
2
3

DOODLE SPACE

LOVING-KINDNESS

TODAYS QUOTABLE

SLEEP SHEETS

BEDTIME: WAKING TIME: APPROX. SLEEP HOURS:

BEDTIME ROUTINE

ACHIEVED
TODAY

1
2
3

MUST DO
TOMORROW

1
2
3

TODAY
I'M GRATEFUL FOR

BRAIN DUMP
AND "DONT FORGETS"

SLEEP HYGINE CHECKS
IF APPLICABLE

1
2
3

DOODLE SPACE

LOVING-KINDNESS

TODAYS QUOTABLE

Sleep Sheets

BEDTIME: WAKING TIME: APPROX. SLEEP HOURS:

BEDTIME ROUTINE

ACHIEVED
TODAY
1.
2.
3.

MUST DO
TOMORROW
1.
2.
3.

TODAY
I'M GRATEFUL FOR

BRAIN DUMP
AND "DONT FORGETS"

SLEEP HYGINE CHECKS
IF APPLICABLE
1.
2.
3.

DOODLE SPACE

LOVING-KINDNESS

TODAYS QUOTABLE

Sleep Sheets

BEDTIME: WAKING TIME: APPROX. SLEEP HOURS:

BEDTIME ROUTINE

ACHIEVED
TODAY

1
2
3

MUST DO
TOMORROW

1
2
3

TODAY
I'M GRATEFUL FOR

BRAIN DUMP
AND "DONT FORGETS"

SLEEP HYGINE CHECKS
IF APPLICABLE

1
2
3

DOODLE SPACE

LOVING-KINDNESS

TODAYS QUOTABLE

SLEEP SHEETS

BEDTIME: WAKING TIME: APPROX. SLEEP HOURS:

BEDTIME ROUTINE

ACHIEVED
TODAY

1
2
3

MUST DO
TOMORROW

1 ○
2 ○
3 ○

TODAY
I'M GRATEFUL FOR

BRAIN DUMP
AND "DONT FORGETS"

SLEEP HYGIENE CHECKS
IF APPLICABLE

1 ○
2 ○
3 ○

DOODLE SPACE

LOVING-KINDNESS

TODAYS QUOTABLE

Sleep Sheets

BEDTIME: WAKING TIME: APPROX SLEEP HOURS:

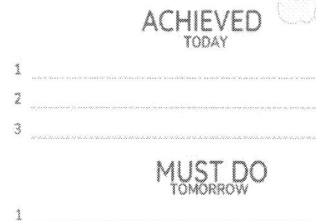

BEDTIME ROUTINE

ACHIEVED
TODAY

1
2
3

MUST DO
TOMORROW

1
2
3

TODAY
I'M GRATEFUL FOR

BRAIN DUMP
AND "DONT FORGETS"

SLEEP HYGINE CHECKS
IF APPLICABLE

1
2
3

DOODLE SPACE

LOVING-KINDNESS

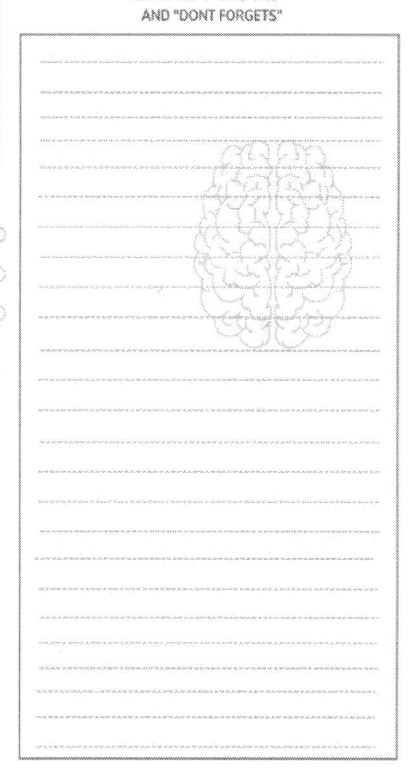

TODAYS QUOTABLE

Sleep Sheets

BEDTIME: WAKING TIME: APPROX. SLEEP HOURS:

BEDTIME ROUTINE

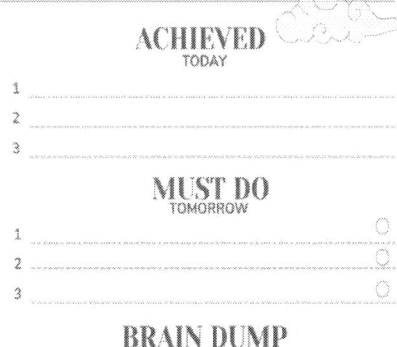

ACHIEVED
TODAY

1
2
3

MUST DO
TOMORROW

1 ○
2 ○
3 ○

TODAY
I'M GRATEFUL FOR

BRAIN DUMP
AND "DONT FORGETS"

SLEEP HYGINE CHECKS
IF APPLICABLE

1 ○
2 ○
3 ○

DOODLE SPACE

LOVING-KINDNESS

TODAYS QUOTABLE

Sleep Sheets

BEDTIME: WAKING TIME: APPROX. SLEEP HOURS:

BEDTIME ROUTINE

ACHIEVED
TODAY
1.
2.
3.

MUST DO
TOMORROW
1. ○
2. ○
3. ○

TODAY
I'M GRATEFUL FOR

BRAIN DUMP
AND "DONT FORGETS"

SLEEP HYGINE CHECKS
IF APPLICABLE
1. ○
2. ○
3. ○

DOODLE SPACE

LOVING-KINDNESS

TODAYS QUOTABLE

Sleep Sheets

BEDTIME: WAKING TIME: APPROX. SLEEP HOURS:

BEDTIME ROUTINE

ACHIEVED
TODAY
1
2
3

MUST DO
TOMORROW
1
2
3

TODAY
I'M GRATEFUL FOR

BRAIN DUMP
AND "DONT FORGETS"

SLEEP HYGINE CHECKS
IF APPLICABLE
1
2
3

DOODLE SPACE

LOVING-KINDNESS

TODAYS QUOTABLE

SLEEP SHEETS

BEDTIME: WAKING TIME: APPROX. SLEEP HOURS:

BEDTIME ROUTINE

ACHIEVED
TODAY
1.
2.
3.

MUST DO
TOMORROW
1.
2.
3.

TODAY
I'M GRATEFUL FOR

BRAIN DUMP
AND "DONT FORGETS"

SLEEP HYGINE CHECKS
IF APPLICABLE
1.
2.
3.

DOODLE SPACE

LOVING-KINDNESS

TODAYS QUOTABLE

Sleep Sheets

BEDTIME: _____   WAKING TIME: _____   APPROX. SLEEP HOURS: _____

BEDTIME ROUTINE

ACHIEVED
TODAY
1.
2.
3.

MUST DO
TOMORROW
1.
2.
3.

TODAY
I'M GRATEFUL FOR

BRAIN DUMP
AND "DONT FORGETS"

SLEEP HYGINE CHECKS
IF APPLICABLE
1.
2.
3.

DOODLE SPACE

LOVING-KINDNESS

TODAYS QUOTABLE

Sleep Sheets

BEDTIME:	WAKING TIME:	APPROX. SLEEP HOURS:

BEDTIME ROUTINE

ACHIEVED
TODAY

1
2
3

MUST DO
TOMORROW

1 ○
2 ○
3 ○

TODAY
I'M GRATEFUL FOR

BRAIN DUMP
AND "DONT FORGETS"

SLEEP HYGINE CHECKS
IF APPLICABLE

1 ○
2 ○
3 ○

DOODLE SPACE

LOVING-KINDNESS

TODAYS QUOTABLE

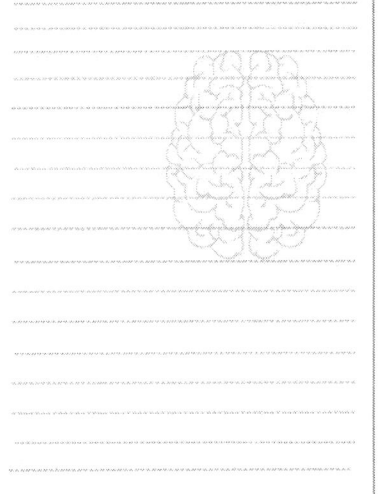

Sleep Sheets

BEDTIME: WAKING TIME: APPROX. SLEEP HOURS:

BEDTIME ROUTINE

ACHIEVED
TODAY
1
2
3

MUST DO
TOMORROW
1
2
3

TODAY
I'M GRATEFUL FOR

BRAIN DUMP
AND "DONT FORGETS"

SLEEP HYGINE CHECKS
IF APPLICABLE
1
2
3

DOODLE SPACE

LOVING-KINDNESS

TODAYS QUOTABLE

Sleep Sheets

BEDTIME: WAKING TIME: APPROX. SLEEP HOURS:

Bedtime Routine

Achieved Today
1.
2.
3.

Must Do Tomorrow
1. ○
2. ○
3. ○

Today I'm Grateful For

Brain Dump
AND "DONT FORGETS"

Sleep Hygine Checks
IF APPLICABLE
1. ○
2. ○
3. ○

Doodle Space

Loving-Kindness

Todays Quotable

SLEEP SHEETS

BEDTIME: WAKING TIME: APPROX. SLEEP HOURS:

BEDTIME ROUTINE

ACHIEVED
TODAY
1
2
3

MUST DO
TOMORROW
1
2
3

TODAY
I'M GRATEFUL FOR

BRAIN DUMP
AND "DONT FORGETS"

SLEEP HYGINE CHECKS
IF APPLICABLE
1
2
3

DOODLE SPACE

LOVING-KINDNESS

TODAYS QUOTABLE

Sleep Sheets

BEDTIME:　　　**WAKING TIME:**　　　**APPROX. SLEEP HOURS:**

BEDTIME ROUTINE

ACHIEVED
TODAY
1
2
3

MUST DO
TOMORROW
1
2
3

TODAY
I'M GRATEFUL FOR

BRAIN DUMP
AND "DONT FORGETS"

SLEEP HYGINE CHECKS
IF APPLICABLE
1
2
3

DOODLE SPACE

LOVING-KINDNESS

TODAYS QUOTABLE

Sleep Sheets

BEDTIME: WAKING TIME: APPROX. SLEEP HOURS:

BEDTIME ROUTINE

ACHIEVED
TODAY

1
2
3

MUST DO
TOMORROW

1
2
3

TODAY
I'M GRATEFUL FOR

BRAIN DUMP
AND "DONT FORGETS"

SLEEP HYGINE CHECKS
IF APPLICABLE

1
2
3

DOODLE SPACE

LOVING-KINDNESS

TODAYS QUOTABLE

Sleep Sheets

BEDTIME: _____ WAKING TIME: _____ APPROX. SLEEP HOURS: _____

BEDTIME ROUTINE

ACHIEVED
TODAY
1. _____
2. _____
3. _____

MUST DO
TOMORROW
1. _____ ○
2. _____ ○
3. _____ ○

TODAY
I'M GRATEFUL FOR

BRAIN DUMP
AND "DONT FORGETS"

SLEEP HYGINE CHECKS
IF APPLICABLE
1. _____ ○
2. _____ ○
3. _____ ○

DOODLE SPACE

LOVING KINDNESS

TODAYS QUOTABLE

Sleep Sheets

BEDTIME: WAKING TIME: APPROX. SLEEP HOURS:

BEDTIME ROUTINE

ACHIEVED
TODAY

1
2
3

MUST DO
TOMORROW

1
2
3

TODAY
I'M GRATEFUL FOR

BRAIN DUMP
AND "DONT FORGETS"

SLEEP HYGINE CHECKS
IF APPLICABLE

1
2
3

DOODLE SPACE

LOVING-KINDNESS

TODAYS QUOTABLE

SLEEP SHEETS

BEDTIME: (WHEN DID YOU GET INTO BED) **WAKING TIME:** (WHEN DID YOU GET UP) **APPROX. SLEEP HOURS:** (FULLY OPTIONAL)

BEDTIME ROUTINE
(LIST WHAT YOU HAVE DONE IN THE PAST 60MINS BEOFRE COMING TO BED E.G. ATE A BISCUIT, READ 4 PAGES OF A BOOK, BRUSHED MY TEETH, FINISHED A MOVIE)

ACHIEVED
TODAY
1. *(THESE DON'T HAVE TO BE HUGE WINS, JUST THINGS THAT*
2. *HAPPENED THAT YOU WOULD LIKE TO KEEP AN EYE ON E.G. WENT*
3. *TO WORK, TOOK A WALK, DID (X) HOBBY, PHONED A FRIEND*

MUST DO
TOMORROW
1. *(HAVE (UPTO) 5 THINGS YOU NEED TO DO TOMORROW".*
2. *PUT THEM HERE AND CHECK THEM OFF TOMORROW*
3. *NIGHT IF YOU LIKE)*

TODAY
I'M GRATEFUL FOR
(NOTE ONE THING THAT WOULD HAVE MADE YOUR DAY WORSE TODAY, HAD YOU NOT HAD IT E.G. SPARE CHANGE FOR THE METER, A TASTY MEAL, A JACKET FOR THE RAINY WEATHER, A BED TO SLEEP IN)

BRAIN DUMP
AND "DONT FORGETS"

IS YOUR BRAIN STILL UP THINKING, START LISTING THINGS HERE, AS THE THOUGHTS COME TO YOU. GREAT PLACE FOR A STREAM OF CONCIOUSNESS, THAT MILLION DOLLAR IDEA YOU HAVE AT 3AM, A REMINDER TO TAKE THE BINS OUT, OR THAT PERFECT COMEBACK FOR THE COWORKER THAT TICKED YOU OFF YESTERDAY

SLEEP HYGINE CHECKS
IF APPLICABLE
1. *(ADD IN AND CHECK OFF ANY PRO-SLEEP BEHAVIOURS YOU ARE WORKING ON DEVELOPING E.G. AVOIDING*
2. *CAFFIENE BEFORE BED, AVOIDING SEDATIVES TO SLEEP, AVOIDING BLUELIGHT/SCREENS 60MIN BEFORE BED,*
3. *BEING PHYSICALY ACTIVE DURING THE DAY, OR GOING TO BED AT A SIMILAR TIME AS YESTERDAY)*

DOODLE SPACE

(A SPACE TO DO A LITTLE DRAWING)

LOVING-KINDNESS
(THINK OF SOMEONE YOU KNOW AND WRITE A WELL INTEDED WISH FOR THEM E.G. I HOPE MY WIFE HAS A GOOD SLEEP, I WISH MY COUSIN LUCK ON THEIR EXAM FINALS NEXT MONTH, I HOPE DAVE FROM PRIMARY SCHOOL IS DOING SOMETHING HE ENJOYS)

TODAYS QUOTABLE
(WHAT IS SOMETHING YOU HEARD, LEARNT, SAID, WROTE TODAY THAT YOU WOULD LIKE TO ABLE TO LOOK BACK ON IN THE FUTURE)

Made in the USA
Columbia, SC
27 May 2023

b6d06b18-b24b-4a6b-858e-05f3c1b91456R01